PATIENT CENTERED MEDICINE

Edited by **Omur Sayligil**

Patient Centered Medicine
http://dx.doi.org/10.5772/63030
Edited by Omur Sayligil

Contributors

Yu Sun, Ana Monteiro Grilo, Balmatee Bidassie, Christopher Kofahl, Alf Trojan, Stefan Nickel, Kenton Stone, Mariel Chance, C.E. Miller, Monika Wahi, Nilüfer Demirsoy, Halil Tekiner, Anne-Sylvie Ramelet, Claire De Labrusse

Published by InTech
Janeza Trdine 9, 51000 Rijeka, Croatia

Publishing Process Manager Romina Skomersic
Technical Editor SPi Global
Cover InTech Design team

First published April, 2017
Printed in Croatia
Legal deposit, Croatia: National and University Library in Zagreb

Additional hard copies can be obtained from orders@intechopen.com

Patient Centered Medicine , Edited by Omur Sayligil
p. cm.
Print ISBN 978-953-51-2991-2
Online ISBN 978-953-51-2992-9

For EU product safety concerns:
IN TECH d.o.o., Prolaz Marije Krucifikse Kozulić 3, 51000 Rijeka, Croatia,
info@intechopen.com or visit our website at intechopen.com.

Meet the editor

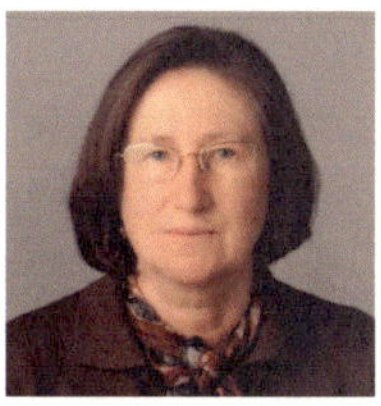

Prof. Dr. Omur Sayligil has been the head of the Department of History of Medicine and Ethics in the Faculty of Medicine at Eskisehir Osmangazi University in Eskisehir, Turkey, since 1994. She completed her bachelor's degree at the Academy of Social Services in Ankara, Turkey (1978), and her Master of Science degrees at the Department of Population Dynamics at Hacettepe University (1981) in Ankara, Turkey, and the Department of Deontology at Uludag University (1987) in Bursa, Turkey. She completed her PhD degree in Deontology and History of Medicine at Ankara University in Ankara, Turkey (1992), on the kidney transplantation from the ethical point of view. She has been working as a professor at the Department of History of Medicine and Ethics in the Faculty of Medicine at Eskisehir Osmangazi University since 2006. She is the author of many articles published in nationally and internationally recognized journals and conference proceedings, and also she contributed to the literature with a number of books and book chapters. Her research interests include medical ethics, organ transplantation, right to live and die, informed consent, research ethics, and ethical committees.

Contents

Preface

Different points of view always existed in medicine. In our age, specialization and healthcare policies are under discussion. Patient-centered medicine is not an illness-centered, a physician-centered, or a hospital-centered medical approach. It cannot be approachedas a surrender to a patients' needs or patients cannot be abandoned to decide on their own after being informed by physicians.. In patient-centered medicine, the patient is evaluated as a whole by taking his/her needs and preferences into account and may discover his/her illness and experience of being ill.

It is possible to define humans from different points of view. Humans, as a certain kind of homotherapeuticus, have aimed at benefiting from treatment opportunities of the time and tried different ways to seek a remedy and utilize resources offered by knowledge and technology through physicians and healthcare professionals, throughout the history. In our age, the latest status of medicine is more about the diseased body, rather than the suffering human.

Development of medical technology, anonymization of patients in medical applications, decrease in patients' self-expression skills, approach to patients as diseases to be treated in hospitals' treatment units, obligation of healthcare professionals to give medical care to a great number of patients in a limited time, lack of empathy of healthcare professionals in a general sense, and certain unethical and illegal actions considered to depend directly on both the people providing and receiving the treatment removed the patients from the center of the medical care, and dehumanization of medicine has come into the picture.

The distance between the patient and physician has been gradually increasing. In spite of the fact that medical services are provided depending on the opportunities and possibilities, damage of communication was previously noticed and emphasized by Hippocrates and, later on, by William Osler. As indicated by W. Osler, "It is much more important to know what sort of a patient has a disease than what sort of a disease a patient has."

In this book, it is aimed at presenting an approach to patient-centered medicine from the beginning of life to the end of life. It may be concluded that the patient-centered approach is a requirement based on humanization of the medicine.

In our day, if the physicians and healthcare professionals could consider more than the diseased organ and provide healthcare by comforting the patients by respecting their values, beliefs, needs, and preferences; informing them and their relatives at every stage; and comforting the patients physically by controlling the pain and relieving their worries and fears, patients obeying the rules of physicians would become patients with high adaptation and participation to the treatment.

Prof. Dr. Omur Sayligil
Eskisehir Osmangazi University
Faculty of Medicine
Eskisehir, Turkey

Chapter 1

Patient-Centred Care in Maternity Services

Claire de Labrusse, Anne Sylvie Ramelet,
Tracy Humphrey and Sara MacLennan

Additional information is available at the end of the chapter

http://dx.doi.org/10.5772/67381

Abstract

Providing patient-centred care (PCC) is one of the goals described by the Institute of Medicine (IOM) to deliver quality of care. Across several interventions described in the literature, there is no clear consensus of one that will best fit the diversity of women coming to seek care in maternity services and across the variety of healthcare providers (HCPs) who provide that care. A reason for that may be the lack of consensus about the model of care to adopt for maternity services reveals a neglected area of research. Managing quality of care should also mean considering the best model of care in practice for all women, incorporating the core and legitimate attributes of maternity care.

Keywords: patient-centred care, maternity services, midwifery, women-centred care, women's health

1. Introduction

Maternity care

Maternity care systems encompass the structures, a diversity of healthcare providers in their expert field of practice and policies that provide antenatal, intrapartum and postnatal care to women and perinatal care to babies. Similar to general health systems, maternity care has evolved over time, but further improvements still need to be made in the future to meet the challenges posed by changing population needs and to increase the involvement of women in their care [1]. The unique feature of maternity services is that the population is predominantly healthy in comparison to other hospital services. Quality of care delivered during pregnancy, labour and the postnatal period refers to the six elements described by the Institute of Medicine (IOM) [2], i.e. (1) safe, (2) effective, (3) patient centred, (4) timely, (5) efficient and

(6) equitable. However, it would be too simplistic to believe that poor quality of care concerns only low- or middle-income countries. For example, in the Mother's Index 2013, it is of note that some high-income regions, such as certain states in the USA, have a higher infant mortality rate than less wealthy countries outside the USA [3, 4].

IOM's quality criteria of safety and effectiveness to improve maternal and foetal outcomes have been a primary target of research for many years [5, 6]. By contrast, patient-centred care (PCC) is just emerging on the maternal and newborn health agenda, and policymakers are only now beginning to address PCC as a dimension of quality of care [7]. The perinatal period is often associated with feelings of anxiety and sometimes even depression [8]. Women across the spectrum of maternity care described the importance of **psychological well-being** and the support received by healthcare providers (HCPs). Anxiety was described in relation to fertility treatment [9], during maternal complications, such as diabetes or high blood pressure [10], when the care was transferred from a midwife to an obstetrician [8], in deprived groups of women [11], or during physiological antenatal, intrapartum and postnatal care[1] [12]. It is important to note that women present various levels of anxiety, regardless of complications or not during the pregnancy. Nevertheless, when anxiety occurred, all women highlighted that continuity by the same HCP or the same group of HCPs (midwives in these articles) helped to build trust and confidence to disclose the origin and the symptoms of anxiety [12].

Women highlighted also the importance of meeting their **care preferences.** In a large questionnaire survey, Baas et al. [8] identified women's desire to receive individualised care as being related to receiving information in a different timeline and through the same HCP. Stevens and Miller [13] linked women's care preferences to the form of communication employed by the HCP, either directive or non-directive. They highlighted that directive information (and not the full options of care) does not meet women's own preferences and specific needs. Similarly, Wickham [14] mentioned how continuity of the HCP was important for many women. This suggests that care should be shaped around women's preferences and needs related to their own values and beliefs. Thus, a directive form of communication with prescriptive information or through the discontinuity of the care provider cannot be considered as responding to women's needs, and a discussion of the subject at an appropriate time is more appreciated and perceived as effective.

By contrast, **communication and information** were highlighted as processes to deliver these components of care. Communication with HCPs was presented as an element to improve the knowledge of the women and to reach a shared decision. How to communicate information was described as the way in which it is possible to influence women's ability to choose between options. Gee and Corry [15] highlighted the importance of women to gain further

[1]This chapter referred to physiological adaptations in pregnancy which are part of the normal process in pregnancy and are mainly in related to (1) cardiovascular, (2) respiratory, (3) renal and (4) biochemical and endocrine changes. Many of these physiological adaptations could be perceived as abnormal in the non-pregnant woman [84]. Pathological conditions during pregnancy are relatively common. The alteration in maternal physiology occurring in pregnancy may affect the pregnancy and the baby [85].

knowledge about their pregnancy and options of care in order to reduce unnecessary tests and interventions. The timing of delivery of information, considered as either too early by some or too late for others, was an issue for the women who did not feel that they had the necessary or individualised information in order to process the situation and make decisions [15, 16]. Furthermore, in a large survey conducted by Attanasio and Kozhimannil [10], women from ethnic minorities (black and Hispanic) addressed having communication issues with HCPs and of being discriminated against because they were uninsured. By contrast, social and deprived groups looked after by a group of midwives (case-load midwifery) expressed their satisfaction with care by their perception of being the centre of attention and building strong relationships with HCPs.

In addition, **case-load midwifery** was highlighted as a process to deliver continuity of care. In her brief report, Wickham revisited the components of continuity of care published by Freeman et al. [17]: (1) management continuity, (2) informational continuity and (3) relationship continuity. Wickham [14] highlighted the importance of the continuity of the HCP as part of a relational continuity. In case-load midwifery, women are allocated to a group of midwives with a primary 'known' midwife, therefore ensuring continuity of carer during the episodes of care. Case-load midwifery was mentioned in several papers reviewed (e.g. a group of midwives [six to eight midwives] who deliver care to a group of women with low and mixed levels of risks at the beginning and during pregnancy, a group of midwives providing antenatal care group sessions to women or groups of midwives for vulnerable women only). In a comparative study of women using case-load midwifery versus standard care, McCourt [18] specifically addressed women's feeling of control and how a strong relationship with the midwife contributed to improve maternal outcomes with fewer interventions during labour (e.g. episiotomy, epidural). Even when complications occurred, the midwife remained a major provider of maternity care and was not withdrawn from care provision. Similar findings were reported [8, 19] who noted the importance of maintaining the named midwife in the continuum of care in relation to psychological well-being, parenting skills and preparation for childbirth. In the physiological context, Overgaard et al. [20] found also that in a freestanding midwifery unit for women with no complications antenatally and during labour, a higher satisfaction of care was reported compared to a traditional labour ward because of the presence of midwives attentive to emotional needs and care preferences.

Therefore, a lack of consensus on the **choice of the model of care** can hinder the further development of quality care. A literature review performed systematically on 'women-centred care' and 'patient-centred care' (five databases searched and additional book review, cross referencing, specialised websites and journals for the search on 'patient-centred care') appraised several models of care for maternity services that were used. Different models of care named were PCC including five to seven domains, women-centred care (WCC), person-centred care, the linguistic model of patient participation in care, centring pregnancy or no model of care. Each model of care has its own definition and focus: (1) PCC encompasses information, communication, emotional support, respect of patient values [20] and 47 standards of outcomes [21]; (2) WCC stated that HCPs should integrate women's preferences and needs into the medical and social characteristics of care [8, 13, 14]; (3) person-centred care was defined with the importance of having someone fully available for them, receiving personalised care, with consistent information [11]; (4) the linguistic model of participation includes the components and processes contributing to patient participation [22]; and (5) centring pregnancy involves a small group of midwives who provide prenatal care to a group of 10–12 women during pregnancy [19]. Wiig et al. [23] highlighted the challenge of using the same definition of quality and its components across the different levels of the systems from micro- and meso- to macro-systems to support quality improvement at all levels of the health systems.

The lack of consensus about the model of care to adopt for maternity services reveals a neglected area of research. Managing quality of care should also mean considering the best model of care in practice for all women, incorporating the core and legitimate attributes of maternity care.

2. Models of care and maternity services?

Women-centred care

One of the most commonly used models within maternity service policies is WCC and is viewed as the cornerstone of the partnership between the midwife and the woman [24–27]. The women-centred philosophy of care emerged after a set of modernising reforms of the NHS and focus on the individualised needs and with the expectation that healthcare professionals would work in collaboration with the women to meet their needs [28]. Within maternity service provision of care, providing WCC would mean that the diversity of HCPs providing maternity care are trained and have the required skills and expertise to meet the women's individual needs.

Women-centred care has been closely linked the midwifery practice, as most of the women have a midwife as their primary health care provider throughout pregnancy, labour and the postnatal period. Whilst the midwife is expert of the care of uncomplicated pregnancies, she also provides a pivotal role in coordinating the journey through pregnancy for all women [29].

The RCM contributed to the developing philosophy of 'woman-centred care' and stated that it is the term used '[for a philosophy of maternity care] that gives priority to the wishes and the needs of the user, and emphasised the importance of informed choice, continuity of care, user involvement, clinical effectiveness, responsiveness and accessibility' ([30], p. 1). The UK and Australian Departments of Health and the Australian College of Midwives also recommend this model of care for maternity services [31–33]. Leap described the wider concept of WCC as a concept that includes the need to address women's emotional, physical, psychological and cultural need and expectations with continuity and control over the care delivered by a single or a group of HCP [34]. This addresses that relationship between the woman and the woman is the key component of the 'women-centred care' which incorporated respectfulness and sensitivity of the midwife [35]. Developing on the idea that WCC was closely linked to midwifery practice, women-centred midwifery was presented by as [36]:

http://dx.doi.org/10.5772/67381

- Focuses on the woman's individual needs, aspirations and expectations, rather than the needs of the institution or professionals
- Recognises the need for women to have choice, control and continuity from a known caregiver or caregivers
- Encompasses the needs of the baby, the woman's family and other people important to the woman, as defined and negotiated by the woman herself
- Follows the woman across the interface of community and acute settings
- Addresses social, emotional, physical, psychological, spiritual and cultural needs and expectations
- Recognises the woman's expertise in decision-making

According to the RCM [37], midwife-led care is the key to achieve a direct link with the defined scope of WCC. The RCM [37] also emphasised that to truly achieve WCC, it needs to be led by midwives through the care they deliver during uncomplicated pregnancies, birth and postnatal care. Similarly, some international definitions of WCC also place an emphasis on uncomplicated pregnancies and normal birth [32, 38]. This has been defined as the care provided by midwives who act as 'the lead professional in the planning, organisation, and delivery of care given to woman (who are healthy and at low risk of complications) from initial booking to the postnatal period' [39]. If, as some professional bodies suggest, midwives can only deliver WCC in the context of uncomplicated childbirth, then it would be exclusive to this discrete group, thus excluding this model of care from a significant and growing proportion of women who have or develop complications or risk factors. However, in the UK, we know that midwives do provide care to *all* women regardless of risk and are often the coordinators of care when there is multidisciplinary/multi-agency involvement. More recently, evidence has shown that WCC has been applied in some services to women who are at high risk of obstetric complications, and there have been demonstrable benefits [28, 40]. This application of WCC reflects the contribution midwives make to women's care despite the care not being *clinically led* by a midwife.

It is estimated that 40% of women are not suitable for midwife-led care at the onset of pregnancy [41], and therefore this proportion of women would not benefit from a WCC model. Furthermore, in clinical situations or countries where healthcare professionals other than midwives are the primary care provider of pregnant women (e.g. family physician or obstetrician), it is not clear whether WCC can be still offered to them [39].

In the process of current identification of WCC, midwifery has been named as being the cornerstone of WCC. In the 1990s, childbirth was becoming 'hypermedicalised', relying more and more on technology, and intervention rates were increasing rapidly and particularly the caesarean section rates. A parliamentary enquiry then determined 'the extent to which resources and professional expertise were used to achieve the most appropriate and cost effective care of pregnant women and delivery and acre of newborn babies'. This was the *Winterton Report*

[42], and the government's response, *Changing Childbirth* [43], recommended more involvement of midwives, development of their roles and greater patient choice over the professional providing care and where to deliver it. So far the government was very focused on mortality rates, but it stressed that the first principle of the maternity service should be 'woman centred'. Policy and professional position papers from the RCM reinforced this association between midwife-led care and WCC.

Fahy [44] wrote an editorial on the definition of WCC in which she argued that midwifery is a discipline that supports the relationship 'with the woman' and that maternity services should support this women-centred midwifery care by providing continuity of relationship during pregnancy and labour. Then, Berg et al. [45] looked at the definition of midwifery care concepts for Sweden and Iceland in the recent literature to identify a midwifery model of WCC that would best fit their context. Their results, as the most current statement about the midwifery care model, addressed that the new midwifery model was similar to the midwifery care model described by the International Confederation of Midwives which gives a focus on normality during pregnancy.

Several projects in Australia and the UK have addressed the importance and the effectiveness of providing WCC for low risk with midwife-led care and high-risk women in collaboration with obstetricians and other HCPs [46, 47]. Leap [34] already addressed the tension that WCC is seen as exclusively linked to normal birth and midwifery-led care [24]. In most circumstances, a midwife would take the role of lead professional for all healthy women with straightforward pregnancies. Additionally, for women with complications, an obstetrician would be the lead professional, and the midwives will provide midwifery care in collaboration with other professionals [41]. The Cochrane review [40] compared midwife-led models of care to other models of care (e.g. obstetrician or family doctor or shared model of care) and suggested that women who received midwife-led models of care were less likely to experience intervention in comparison with women who received other models of care. The review included studies with women classified as both 'high and low' risk, with the exclusion of women currently experiencing both acute maternal complication and substance misuse. The authors note that the same results may not be applicable with women experiencing obstetrical complications and not being under midwife-led care. It is only recently that the RCOG have embraced this concept in their guidelines. In the revised position statement in 2008, the RCM stipulated that "truly WCC must encompass midwifery-led care of normal pregnancy, birth and the postnatal period and services that are planned and delivered close to women and the communities in which they live or work." ([37], p. 2). This statement highlights WCC as including uncomplicated pregnancy, with midwife-led care being provided in midwife-led settings such as home, freestanding and alongside hospital birth centres for women defined as having a low clinical risk.

Finally, the key concepts of quality in maternal and newborn care presented in the Lancet Midwifery [48] included: safe, effective, accessible, appropriate, affordable, equitable, efficient, and woman-centred care. This framework for maternal and newborn care referenced the WHO Quality of Care report [49] as the primary reference, but they use the term patient-centred care not women-centred care, which highlights one example of the terms PCC and

http://dx.doi.org/10.5772/67381

WCC not being used consistently. This may be due to a lack of clarity about their dimensions and in which context one should be used and not in the other. The results of this study have highlighted the gaps in WCC as needing to be more inclusive of women, regardless of risk or model of care. Until there is more consistency and acceptance about WCC for all women, regardless of model of care, it may be that, as this study suggests that PCC may be a more inclusive model.

More recently, contemporary policy documents have alluded to WCC being for all women—not just those receiving midwife-led care [50, 51]. If WCC is to apply to all women using maternity services, then it would be beneficial to reflect this in its definition. For example, specifying that WCC is for all women, regardless of risk, pathway of care or lead healthcare professional. This would be more inclusive and support maternity services to apply this concept more broadly, enabling all women to benefit from this philosophy of care.

Identifying the most appropriate model of care for maternity services with a clear definition of each domain would help governments and professionals to develop goals and implementation strategies to improve the quality of care delivered. The review of other models used in maternity service policies shows that family-centred care places an emphasis on the sick child [52, 53] and person-centred care relates mainly to elderly people or those with long-term health conditions [54, 55]. Thus, these last two terms do not match the state of health and age of women in their reproductive life using maternity services [56]. Therefore, an alternative model of care is necessary for women who present various status of health when being pregnant. PCC has also been used in maternity service policies and offers such an alternative [57–59].

3. Reflection on Shaller's PCC model and redefinition [60]

PCC has been recommended as a marker of quality in health service delivery [61]. There are numerous definitions of PCC, but one of the most influential models that formed the foundation of the PCC approach was developed by Gerteis et al. [62] for the Picker Institute and incorporates seven key domains: (1) respect for patient values, preferences and expressed needs; (2) coordination and integration of care; (3) information, communication and education; (4) physical comfort; (5) emotional support and alleviation of fear and anxiety; (6) involvement of family and friends; and (7) transition and continuity.

Whereas other models may not be inclusive of the diversity of care that women may need, the 'coordination and integration of care' domain of the PCC model encompasses various care pathways that can fit with the uncertainty of childbirth. Of note, this domain is not dependent on the HCP function and incorporates the variety of healthcare professionals that some women may encounter, including the dynamic nature of risk within pregnancy. This has the advantage to allow women to easily transit from one pathway of care to another without any effect on their model of care. Finally, the PCC 'respect for patient values, preferences and expressed needs' domain is comprehensive enough to consider the general and specific issues of women's needs and expectations when using maternity services. When one of the most referenced definitions of PCC is reviewed, it appears that PCC may be a more appropriate model of care for maternity services, as per described; see [63]. Shaller's [60] framework of PCC described a brief outline of the six domains including:

- Domain 1: Education and shared knowledge
- Domain 2: Involvement of family and friends
- Domain 3: Collaboration and team management
- Domain 4: Sensitivity to non-medical and spiritual dimensions
- Domain 5: Respect for patient need and preferences
- Domain 6: Free-flow and accessibility of information

A comparison of the data collected in the multiple case study approach about maternity services with the existing literature highlighted further elements in each one of the domains. A revised model could integrate a stronger appreciation of the importance to provide individualised information by their care provider (d1), highlighting the opportunity for a greater involvement of the family and friends (d2), with a continuity of care (d3), an awareness of anxiety in any pregnancies and the midwife as the person to refer to in this situation (d4), and the development of clear and achievable expectations (d5), using multiple interventions that support communication. A revised model of PCC presented below is inspired by the Shaller definitions (plain text) and includes additional or alternative terms about the domains. This revised model provides more details and uses semantics that are generalisable to other services not just for maternity services but also for other health areas.

4. Proposed revised model of PCC

Domain 1: Timely, complete (generic and individual), evidence-based information that would be delivered by experts in the field (ideally their care provider). This information should reflect the diverse opportunities made available to women by the institution to be involved in care delivery (antenatal consultation, antenatal classes, hand-held records, diaries, private consultations, etc.).

Domain 2: Involvement of partner and family in decision-making as an advocate of the woman when needed and with an awareness and accommodation of their needs as caregivers with an evaluation of their experience as service users.

Domain 3: Continuity of care between the diverse HCPs and the person receiving the care, with the inclusion of their partner and family during physiological and complicated care.

Domain 4: Incorporating emotional support, spirituality and attention to non-pharmaceutical treatments (e.g. human touch, massage, etc.), with an awareness of quality of life.

Domain 5: Respect of patient's needs, preferences, beliefs and values. Supporting people to develop achievable aims and to know also what they can expect from the institution.

Domain 6: Informing and empowering patients through consumer-oriented health libraries and patient education. Healthcare practitioners communicate and share complete and unbiased information with patients and families using diverse strategies freely accessible outside the hospital and out-of-normal hours.

5. Relating the revised model to existing literature

The proposed revised definitions of PCC are close to the person-centred care definition published by the Scottish government in the Healthcare Quality Strategy for NHS Scotland (2010) and so beyond the disease-oriented definition, including shared decision-making and mutual partnership with the person and their families.

It became apparent that policies were shifting their terminology from PCC in those reviewed after 2009 [64–70] to person-centred care in the last policy analysed [71]. Over the past 5 years, the model of person centredness has increasingly appeared in UK health policy and, more specifically, in Scotland in the past 5 years. Today, person-centred care is also central to the four UK countries, i.e. Vision 2020 for Scotland [72], the Health and Social Care Act [73], Department of Health Northern Ireland [74], and the Welsh White Paper [75]. Whereas prior PCC definitions focused on the pathology [2, 76] and the person-centred model on oncological and gerontological care [55, 77], the recent definitions of person-centred care by the Health Foundation [54] have tried to include principles, rather than a definition, for example:

'(1) Affording people dignity, compassion and respect. (2) Offering coordinated care, support or treatment. (3) Offering personalised care, support or treatment. (4) Supporting people to recognise and develop their own strengths and abilities to enable them to live an independent and fulfilling life' ([54], p. 6).

The Health Foundation proposed four principles of person-centred care rather than definitions as they can be restrictive. Unfortunately, it omitted to explain how each one of the principles could be delivered in practice, which can be more easily evaluated and improved upon than proposing broad approaches that are not clearly linked to one principle. The levels of the principles do not yet provide the level of details that Shaller's model proposes, which supports a clearer implementation and evaluation process. Through this research the Shaller's model has been demonstrated to be appropriate for maternity services as it offers a model of care that includes a continuum from wellness to illness for women who present in various states of health during the course of their pregnancy. The similarities of the themes used between PCC and person-centred care (e.g. respect, support and positive reinforcement) and between PCC and WCC (e.g. individual needs (emotional, physical, psychological, spiritual), choice, continuity and decision) provide evidence of PCC's relevance and potential. The research also demonstrates how this could be further improved.

A clear definition of the model of care is essential for policymakers and practitioners to improve the system in place. Giving a definition of the PCC model in the policy will help the implementation of the intervention and set the scene for its evaluation and the further revision of the policy and the model itself [78]. Clarity and transparency of the model of care chosen and its accompanying definition will benefit its implementation along the whole pathway [79]. To date, Shaller's theoretical framework appears to be the most inclusive model and remains the representation of PCC reported at global level. The domains have also recently been used in describing person-centred care [80–83]. It could be because its definitions and key factors for achieving PCC are the most representative to complex health systems, with the acknowledgement that no other theoretical framework has been able to address both the diversity of women's clinical conditions and HCPs' provision of roles.

Author details

Claire de Labrusse[1*], Anne Sylvie Ramelet[2], Tracy Humphrey[3] and Sara MacLennan[4]

*Address all correspondence to: Claire.delabrusse@hesav.ch

1 University of Health Sciences Western Switzerland (HESAV), Lausanne, Switzerland

2 Institut Universitaire de formation et de recherche en soins-IUFRS University of Lausanne, Lausanne, Switzerland

3 Edinburgh Napier University, School of Health & Social Care, Edinburgh, Scotland

4 Academic Urology Unit, University of Aberdeen, Aberdeen, Scotland

References

[1] Malatest International Consulting and Advisory Service. Comparative study of maternity services. 2012. Available from: https://www.health.govt.nz/system/files/documents/publications/comparative-study-of-maternity-systems-nov13.pdf [Accessed 11 April 2016].

[2] Institute of Medicine (IOM). Crossing the quality chasm: a new health system for the 21th Century. Washington, D.C.: National Academies Press. 2001. 337 p.

[3] MacDorman M F, Matthews T J, Mohangoo A D, Zeitlin J. International comparisons of infant mortality and related factors: United States and Europe, 2010. National Vital Statistics Report. 2014; **63**(5): 1–6.

[4] Save the Children. State of the world's mothers: the urban disadvantage. 2015. Available from: https://www.savethechildren.net/state-worlds-mothers-2015 [Accessed 11 April 2016].

[5] Souza J P, Gülmezoglu A M, Vogel J, Carroli G, Lumbiganon P, Qureshi Z, Costa M J, Fawole B, Mugerwa Y, Nafiou I, Neves I, Wolomby-Molondo J J, Bang H, Cheang K, Chuyun K, Jayaratne K, Jayathilaka C, Mazhar S, Mori R, Mustafa M, Pathak L, Rathavy T, Recidoro Z, Roy M, Ruyan P, Shrestha N, Taneepanichsku S, Tien N, Ganchimeg T,

Wehbe M, Yadamsuren B, Yan W, Yunis K, Bataglia V, Cecatti J, Hernandez-Prado B, Nardin J, Narváez A, Ortiz-Panozo E, Pérez-Cuevas R, Valladares E, Zavaleta N, Armson A, Crowther C, Hogue C, Lindmark G, Mittal S, Pattinson R, Stanton M, Campodonico L, Cuesta C, Giordano D, Intarut N, Laopaiboon M, Bahl R, Martines J, Mathai M, Merialdi M, Say L. Moving beyond essential interventions for reduction of maternal mortality (the WHO multicountry survey on maternal and newborn health): a cross-sectional study. Lancet. 2013; **381**(9879): 1747–1755.

[6] World Health Organization, World Bank, United Nations Fund for Population Activities, United Nations International Children's Emergency Fund. Trends in maternal mortality: 1990 to 2015. Geneva: WHO. 2015. Available from: http://www.who.int/reproductivehealth/publications/monitoring/maternal-mortality-2015/en/ [Accessed 12 April 2016].

[7] Van Lerberghe W, Matthews Z, Achadi E, Ancona C, Campbell J, Channon A, de Bernis L, De Brouwere V, Fauveau V, Fogstad H, Koblinsky M, Liljestrand J, Mechbal A, Murray S F, Rathavay T, Rehr H, Richard F, ten Hoope-Bender P, Turkmani S. Country experience with strengthening of health systems and deployment of midwives in countries with high maternal mortality. Lancet. 2014; **384**(9949): 1215–1225.

[8] Baas C I, Erwich JJ, Wiegers T A, de Cock T P, Hutton E K. Women's suggestions for improving midwifery care in The Netherlands. Birth. 2015; **42**(4): 369–378.

[9] Aarts J W, Huppelschoten A G, van Empel I W, Boivin J, Verhaak C M, Kremer JA, Nelen W L. How patient-centred care relates to patients' quality of life and distress: a study in 427 women experiencing infertility. Human Reproduction. 2012; **27**(2): 488–495.

[10] Attanasio L, Kozhimannil K B. Patient-reported communication quality and perceived discrimination in maternity care. Medical Care Journal. 2015; **53**(10): 863–871.

[11] Beake S, Acosta L, Cooke P, McCourt C. Caseload midwifery in a multi-ethnic community: the women's experiences. Midwifery. 2013; **29**(8): 996–1002.

[12] Frei A, Mander R. The relationship between first-time mothers and care providers in the early postnatal phase: an ethnographic study in a Swiss postnatal unit. Midwifery. 2011; **27**(5): 716–722

[13] Stevens G, Miller Y D. Overdue Choices: How Information and Role in Decision-Making Influence Women's Preferences for Induction for Prolonged Pregnancy. Birth. 2012; **39**(3): 248–257.

[14] Wickham S. Being clear about continuity. Practicing Midwife. 2015; **18**(7): 42–43

[15] Gee R, Corry M. Patient engagement and shared decision making in maternity care. Obstetrics & Gynaecology. 2012; **120**(5): 995–997.

[16] Cheyne H, McCourt C, Semple K. Mother knows best: developing a consumer led, evidence informed, research agenda for maternity care. Midwifery. 2013; **29**(6): 705–712.

[17] Freeman G K, Woloshynowych M, Boulton M, Guthrie B, Car J, Haggerty J, Tarrant C. Continuity of care 2006: what have we learned since 2000 and what are policy imperatives now? Report for the National Co-ordinating Centre for NHS service delivery and organisation R & D (NCCSDO), London, UK: NCCSDO. 2007. Available from: http://www.netscc.ac.uk/hsdr/files/project/SDO_FR_08-1609-138_V01.pdf [Accessed 23 May 2016]

[18] McCourt C. Technologies of birth and models of midwifery care. Revista da Escola de Enfermagem. 2014; **48**(suppl.): 168–177.

[19] McNeil J A, Reiger K M. Rethinking prenatal care within a social model of health: an exploratory study in Northern Ireland. Health Care Women International. 2015; **36**(1): 5–25.

[20] Overgaard C, Fenger-Gron M, Sandal, J. The impact of birthplace on women's birth experiences and perceptions of care. Social Science Medicine. 2012; 74(7): 973–981.

[21] Moore J E, Titler M G, Kane Low L, Dalton V K, Sampselle C M. Transforming patient-centered care: development of the evidence informed decision making through engagement model. Women's Health Issues. 2015; 25(3): 276–282.

[22] Heatley M L, Watson B, Gallois C, Miller Y D. Women's perceptions of communication in pregnancy and childbirth: influences on participation and satisfaction with care. Journal of Health Communication. 2015; 20(7): 827–834.

[23] Wiig S, Aase K, von Plessen C, Burnett S, Nunes F, Weggelaar A M, Anderson-Gare B, Calltorp J, Fulop N, Quaser TeamTalking about quality: exploring how 'quality' is conceptualized in European hospitals and healthcare systems. BMC Health Services Research. 2014; **14**: 478.

[24] Carolan M, Hodnett E. 'With woman' philosophy: examining the evidence, answering the questions. Nursing Inquiry. 2007; **14**(2): 140–152.

[25] Hodnett E D. Continuity of caregivers for care during pregnancy and childbirth. Cochrane Database of Systematic Reviews. 2000; 2, CD000062.

[26] Hodnett E D. Pain and women satisfaction with the experience of childbirth: a systematic review. American Journal of Obstetrics and Gynaecology. 2002; **186**: 160–172.

[27] Moscucci O. Holistic obstetrics: the origins of "natural childbirth" in Britain. Postgraduate Medicine Journal. 2003; **79**(929): 168–173.

[28] Pope R, Graham L, Patel S. Woman-centred care. International Journal of Nursing Studies. 2001; **38**(2): 227–238.

[29] NHS Education for Scotland (NES). Midwifery 2020 Programme. Core role of the Midwife Workstream Final Report. 2010. Available from: http://www.nes.scot.nhs.uk/media/1891153/core_role.pdf. [Accessed 10 July 2016]

[30] Royal College of Midwives (RCM). Position paper No. 4a. Woman-centred care. London, UK: RCM. 2001.

[31] Department of Health. National Service Framework for Children, Young People and Maternity Services. 2004. Available from: https://www.gov.uk/government/uploads/system/uploads/attachment_data/file/199952/National_Service_Framework_for_Children_Young_People_and_Maternity_Services_-_Core_Standards.pdf [Accessed 10 April 2016].

[32] Department of Health New South Wales (Australia). Maternity—towards normal birth in NSW. 2010. Available from: http://www0.health.nsw.gov.au/policies/pd/2010/pdf/PD2010_045.pdf [Accessed 10 April 2016].

[33] Australian College of Midwives. 2011. ACM philosophy for midwifery. Available from: http://www.midwives.org.au/scripts/cgiip.exe/WService=MIDW/ccms.r?pageid=10019 [Accessed 8 April 2016].

[34] Leap E. Women-centred care or women centred care: does it matter? British Journal of Midwifery. 2009; **17**(1): 12–16.

[35] Page L. Effective group practice in midwifery: working with women. Oxford [England]; Cambridge, Mass. USA: Blackwell Science. 1995.

[36] Leap, N. 'The less we do, the more we give'. Basingstoke: Macmillan. 2000.

[37] Royal College of Midwives (RCM). Position statement—Woman-centred care. London, UK: RCM. 2008.

[38] American College of Nurses and Midwives (ACNM). Core values ACNM. 2014. Available from: http://www.midwife.org/Our-Mission-Vision-Values [Accessed 8 April 2016].

[39] Sandall J, Soltani H, Gates S, Shennan A, Devane D. Midwife-led continuity models versus other models of care for childbearing women (review). Cochrane Database of Systematic Reviews. 2013. **3**(8): 3.

[40] Sandall J, Soltani H, Gates S, Shennan A, Devane D. Midwife-led continuity models versus other models of care for childbearing women. Cochrane Database of Systematic Reviews. 2015. Issue 9.

[41] Royal College of Midwives (RCM). The Royal College of Midwives' audit of midwifery practice. London, UK: RCM. 2010. Available from: https://www.rcm.org.uk/sites/default/files/Practice%20Full%20ReportAug2011FINAL_0.pdf [Accessed 11 April 2016].

[42] House of Commons. The health Committee Second Report: Maternity Services. London. HMSO. 1992.

[43] Department of Health. Changing Childbirth, Part I: Report of the Expert Maternity Group. London. HMSO. 1993.

[44] Fahy K. What is woman-centred care and why does it matter? Women and Birth. 2012; **25**(4): 149–151.

[45] Berg M, Ólafsdóttir Ó A, Lundgren I. A midwifery model of woman-centred childbirth care–in Swedish and Icelandic settings. Sexual & Reproductive Healthcare. 2012; **3**(2): 79–87.

[46] North Staffordshire Changing Childbirth Research Team. A randomised study of midwifery caseload care and traditional 'shared-care'. Midwifery. 2000; **16**(4): 295–302.

[47] Tracy S K, Hartz D L, Tracy M B, Allen J, Forti A, Hall B, White J, Lainchbury A, Stapleton H, Beckmann M, Bisits A, Homer C, Foureur M, Welsh A, Kildea S. Caseload midwifery care versus standard maternity care for women of any risk: M@NGO, a randomised controlled trial. Lancet; 2013; **382**(9906): 1723–1732. doi: 10.1016/s0140-6736(13)61406-3

[48] Renfrew M J, McFadden A, Bastos M H, Campbell J, Channon A A, Cheung N F, Declercq E. Midwifery and quality care: findings from a new evidence-informed framework for maternal and newborn care. Lancet. 2014; **384**(9948): 1129–1145.

[49] World Health Organization. Quality of care. A process for making strategies choices in health systems. 2006. Available at: http://www.who.int/management/quality/assurance/QualityCare_B.Def.pdf?ua=1 [Accessed 17 October 2016]

[50] Royal College of Midwives (RCM). High quality Midwifery care. 2014. Available from: https://www.rcm.org.uk/sites/default/files/High%20Quality%20Midwifery%20Care%20Final.pdf [Accessed 5 September 2016]

[51] National Health Service England. (2015). National Review of Maternity Services: Assessment of Quality in Maternity Services. Retrieved from https://www.england.nhs.uk/wp-content/uploads/2015/07/Assessment-of-Quality-in-Maternity-Services.pdf [Accessed 9 May 2016]

[52] Shields L, Pratt J, Hunter J. Family centred care: a review of qualitative studies. Journal of Clinical Nursing. 2006; **15**(10): 1317–1323.

[53] Svavarsdottir E K. Listening to the family's voice: Nordic nurses' movement toward family centered care. Journal of Family Nursing. 2006; **12**(4): 346–367

[54] Health Foundation. Person-centred care made simple. London, UK: Health Foundation. 2014. Available from http://www.health.org.uk/sites/default/files/PersonCentredCareMadeSimple.pdf [Accessed 11 April 2016].

[55] Victorian Government Department of Human Services. What is person-centred health care? A literature review. National Ageing Research Institute, State Government of Victoria, Australia. 2006. Available from: http://www.mednwh.unimelb.edu.au/pchc/downloads/PCHC_literature_review.pdf [Accessed 12 April 2016].

[56] Travis J W, Ryan RS. Wellness workbook: How to achieve enduring health and vitality (3rd ed.). Berkeley, CA: Celestial Arts. 2004.

[57] Australian Commission on Safety and Quality in Health Care. National Safety and Quality Health Service Standard 2: Partnering with consumers – embedding partnerships in health care. 2014. Available from: http://www.safetyandquality.gov.au/wp-content/uploads/2014/11/Partnering-with-Consumers-Embedding-partnerships-in-health-care.pdf [Accessed 10 April 2016].

[58] Docteur E, Coulter A. Patient-centredness in Sweden's health system. An assessment and six steps for progress. 2012. Swedish Agency for Health and Care Services Analysis, Stockholm.

[59] Ministry of Health British Columbia. Enabling effective, quality population and patient-centred care: a provincial strategy for health human resources. Victoria, BC, Canada: Ministry of Health. 2015. Available from: http://www.health.gov.bc.ca/library/publications/year/2015/health-human-resources-policy-paper.pdf [Accessed 11 April 2016].

[60] Shaller D. Patient-centered care: what does it take?. New York/Washington, D.C: The Commonwealth Fund. 2007. Available from: http://www.commonwealthfund.org/usr_doc/Shaller_patient-centeredcarewhatdoesittake_1067.pdf?section=4039 [Accessed 11 April 2016].

[61] Scottish Executive Health Department. Better health, better care. Discussion document. Edinburgh: NHS Scotland. 2007. Available from: http://www.gov.scot/resource/doc/194854/0052337.pdf [Accessed 27 April 2016]

[62] Gerteis M, Edgman-Levitan S, Daley J, Delbanco LT. Through the patient's eye. New York: Jossey-Bass. 1993.

[63] De Labrusse C, Ramelet A S, Humphrey T, Maclennan S J. Patient-centered care in maternity services: a critical appraisal and synthesis of the literature. Women's Health Issues. 2016; **26**(1): 100–109.

[64] Scottish Government. Expert group on acute maternity services. Edinburgh: Scottish Executive. 2002. Available from: http://www.gov.scot/Publications/2003/01/16018/15751 [Accessed 11 April 2016].

[65] Scottish Government. Delivering for health. Edinburgh: Scottish Executive. 2005. Available from: http://www.gov.scot/resource/doc/76169/0018996.pdf [Accessed 11 April 2016].

[66] Scottish Executive Health Department. National framework for service change in NHS Scotland. (The Kerr report). Edinburgh: NHS Scotland. 2005. Available from: http://www.sehd.scot.nhs.uk/nationalframework/ [Accessed 27 April 2016]

[67] Scottish Government. Delivering care, enabling health: harnessing the nursing, midwifery and allied health professions' contribution to implementing delivering for health in Scotland. Edinburgh: Scottish Executive. 2006. Available from: http://www.gov.scot/resource/doc/152499/0041001.pdf [Accessed 11 April 2016].

[68] Scottish Government. Better health, better care: action plan. Edinburgh: Scottish Executive. 2007. Available from: http://www.gov.scot/Resource/Doc/206458/0054871.pdf [Accessed 11 April 2016].

[69] Scottish Government. CURAM nurses, midwives and allied health professionals working for Scotland's health. Edinburgh: Scottish Executive. 2009. Available from: http://www.gov.scot/resource/doc/254463/0075344.pdf [Accessed 11 April 2016].

[70] Scottish Government. Health care quality strategy. Edinburgh: Scottish Executive. 2010. Available from: http://www.gov.scot/resource/doc/311667/0098354.pdf [Accessed 11 April 2016].

[71] Scottish Government. A refreshed framework for maternity care in Scotland. The maternity services action group. Edinburgh: Scottish Executive. 2011. Available from: http://www.gov.scot/Resource/Doc/341632/0113609.pdf [Accessed 11 April 2016].

[72] Scottish Government. Everyone matters: 2020 workforce vision. Edinburgh: Scottish Executive. 2013. Available from: http://www.gov.scot/resource/0042/00424225.pdf [Accessed 11 April 2016].

[73] United Kingdom Parliament. Health and Social Care Act 2012, c.7. 2012. Available from: http://www.legislation.gov.uk/ukpga/2012/7/contents/enacted [Accessed 11 April 2016].

[74] Department of Health Northern Ireland. Northern Ireland 2020 Quality Strategy. Safety and Quality Standard, 2020. Department of Health. 2011. Available from: https://www.health-ni.gov.uk/publications/quality-2020-ten-year-strategy-protect-and-improve-quality-health-and-social-care. [Accessed 28 May 2016]

[75] Welsh Government. Welsh White paper. Legislative proposal for additional learning needs. Welsh Government: Cardiff. 2014. Available from: http://dera.ioe.ac.uk/20172/1/140522-consultation-document-en.pdf. [Accessed 17 October 2016]

[76] Richards N, Coulter A. "Is the NHS becoming more patient-centred? Trends from the national surveys of NHS patients in England 2002-07." 2007. Available from http://www.pickereurope.org/Filestore/PIE_reports/project_reports/Trends_with_ISBN_web_(3).pdf.

[77] Health Foundation. Person-centred care: from ideas to action. Health Foundation. 2014. Available from: http://www.health.org.uk/sites/default/files/PersonCentredCareFromIdeasToAction.pdf [Accessed 11 April 2016].

[78] Mazmanian D A, Sabatier P A. Implementation and public policy: with a new postscript. Lanham/New York/London: University Press of America. 1989.

[79] Van Meter D S, Van Horn C E. The policy implementation process: a conceptual framework. Administration & Society. 1975; **6**(4): 445–488.

[80] Luxford K, Safran D G, Delbanco T. Promoting patient-centered care: a qualitative study of facilitators and barriers in healthcare organizations with a reputation for improving the patient experience. International Journal for Quality in Health Care. 2011; **23**(5): 510–515.

[81] Adams M, Maben J, Robert G. Improving patient-centred care through experience-based co-design (EBCD): an evaluation of the sustainability and spread of EBCD in a cancer centre. King's College. London. 2014.

[82] Baker G R. Evidence boost: A review of research highlighting how patient engagement contributes to improved care. 2014. Available from: http://www.cfhi-fcass.ca/sf-docs/default-source/reports/evidenceboost-rossbaker-peimprovedcare-e.pdf?sfvrsn=8 [Accessed 28 May 2016]

http://dx.doi.org/10.5772/67381

[83] Picker Institute. Person-centred care in Europe: a cross-country comparison of health system performance, strategies and structures. 2016. Available from: http://www.pickereurope.org/wp-content/uploads/2016/02/12-02-16-Policy-briefing-on-patient-centred-care-in-Europe.pdf. [Accessed 28 May 2016]

[84] Hoffman, B. L. & Williams, J. M. Williams obstetrics. 2014. London : McGraw-Hill Education.

[85] Magowan, B., Owen, P., Thompson, A. Clinical obstetrics and gynaecology. 2014. Edinburgh; New York, Saunders.

Chapter 2

Patient-Centered Medicine and Prevention of Munchausen Syndrome by Proxy

Monika M. Wahi, Kenton V. Stone,
Mariel Chance and Cynthia E. Miller

Additional information is available at the end of the chapter

http://dx.doi.org/10.5772/65814

Abstract

Munchausen syndrome by proxy (MSbP) is known by many names and is considered the deadliest form of child abuse. Although the condition was named in 1976 and there is now a substantial body of scientific literature about this type of abuse, to date, patient-centered approaches to early identification, intervention, and prevention have been absent from this literature. The purpose of this chapter is to recommend patient-centered approaches to identifying MSbP in the clinical setting to facilitate prevention and early intervention. It also recommends patient-centered practices that can be implemented to reduce the MSbP-related morbidity and mortality contributed by the healthcare system. The evolving nomenclature and definition of MSbP abuse has been an obstacle to achieving scientific consensus on the topic. Yet, the body of scientific literature on the subject is large. This literature is reviewed to enumerate the healthcare system's contribution to MSbP abuse. The Haddon matrix, a public health framework, is applied to MSbP abuse in order to guide the development of recommendations of patient-centered approaches that should be implemented to reduce the healthcare system's contribution to the morbidity and mortality that MSbP victims face.

Keywords: Munchausen syndrome by proxy, public health practice, delivery of health care, child abuse, malpractice

1. Introduction

Munchausen syndrome by proxy (MSbP) is known by many names and is considered the deadliest form of child abuse. Although the condition was named in 1976 and there is now a substantial body of scientific literature about this type of abuse, to date, patient-centered approaches to early identification, intervention, and prevention have been absent from this literature. In the discussion of this condition, there has been a particular lack of emphasis on the role of the healthcare system in this abuse.

This chapter summarizes the research on MSbP and recommends patient-centered approaches to identifying MSbP in the clinical setting to facilitate prevention and early intervention. It also recommends patient-centered practices that can be implemented to reduce the MSbP-related morbidity and mortality contributed by the healthcare system. The first section of this chapter explains the evolving nomenclature and definition of MSbP abuse. The second section reviews the scientific literature to enumerate the healthcare system's contribution to MSbP abuse. Finally, this chapter applies a public health framework to MSbP abuse in order to recommend patient-centered approaches that should be implemented to reduce the health-care system's contribution to the morbidity and mortality that MSbP victims face.

2. Understanding the nature of MSbP

This section reviews the history of thought on the condition this chapter will refer to as MSbP, which is recognized as the deadliest form of child abuse [1], although it is acknowledged that other names have been used. First, this section covers initial identification of the condition and early attempts to name and define it. Next, this section discusses the evolution of diagnostic criteria for MSbP. Third, the challenges to studying MSbP victims are covered, and after that, challenges to developing a public health perspective on MSbP are outlined. Finally, a novel patient-centered perspective on MSbP abuse is proposed to facilitate early identification, early effective intervention, and the possibility of prevention of MSbP abuse in the healthcare system.

2.1. The evolution of names of MSbP

Currently, there is no agreed-upon definition of MSbP, though MSbP is believed to be the cause of most deaths initially attributed to sudden infant death syndrome (SIDS), which has now been debunked as an actual disease entity[1] [1, 4–7]. Though the condition was originally named MSbP in 1976 by British pediatrician Roy Meadow [8], the condition had previously been defined in the literature under other disease entities, such as "non-accidental poisoning" [9] or "maltreatment syndrome" [10].

Clinicians and researchers struggled to separate this condition from other conditions, because the main symptoms identified at the time were (1) a guardian of a child (generally the mother) fabricating or inducing illness in a child to obtain unneeded medical care for the child and (2) abnormal personality characteristics in the perpetrating guardian [8]. The fact that at least two people were involved in this syndrome, the perpetrator and the child victim, made it difficult to define. Child advocates used names that focused on the child abuse aspect of the condition

[1]Although currently, for whatever reason, scientific writers and public health advocates do not appear to acknowledge that SIDS is not an entity and is instead a likely case of MSbP, as evidenced by Refs. [2] and [3].

http://dx.doi.org/10.5772/65814

[11, 12], while psychologists were more interested in establishing and naming a mental health diagnosis for the perpetrator [13–15].

This early division in approach to this syndrome creates confusion in the scientific literature to this day. Although the literature has coalesced around the term MSbP, other terms are still used, confounding efforts to assemble a historical scientific picture of the evolution of understanding this condition. Terms used in history as well as today for this syndrome include Polle syndrome [16, 17], terms that include the word "factitious" such as "factitious disorder by proxy" [18–21], "illness induction" [22, 23], and more recently, "medical child abuse" [24, 25]. Scientific writers struggled to find the right term to use [26–30] and also with "who" was being diagnosed with the disorder – the child victim, the perpetrator, the duo together, or the entire family [31, 32].

2.2. Diagnostic criteria for MSbP

Attempts to establish diagnostic criteria have been fraught with dissention. In 1995, Meadow proposed the following criteria, all of which would have to be met to assign a positive diagnosis: (1) Illness in a child which is fabricated by a parent, or someone who is in *loco parentis* (acting in the role of a parent of a child), (2) the child is presented for medical assessment and care, usually persistently, often resulting in multiple medical procedures, (3) the perpetrator denies the etiology of the child's illness, and (4) acute symptoms and signs of illness cease when the child is separated from the perpetrator [33]. The third item has been a focus of psychologists interested in studying the perpetrator, as it has been noted that perpetrators caught on video surveillance engaging in MSbP behaviors may continue to deny their involvement [34]. The fourth item has been hotly debated, as victims who have been severely injured by MSbP abuse may not have their acute symptoms and signs of illness cease because real damage has been done as the result of the abuse [35].

In 2003, Rosenberg proposed the following diagnostic criteria for MSbP, of which all must be met in order to assign a positive diagnosis: (1) Child has been repeatedly presented for medical care, (2) test/event is positive for tampering with child, or with child's medical situation, (3) positivity of test/event is not credibly the result of test error or misinterpretation, nor of miscommunication or of specimen handling, (4) no explanation for the positive test/event other than illness falsification is medically possible, and (5) no findings credibly exclude illness falsification [36]. Unlike Meadow's criteria, these focus on confirming that the perpetrator is manipulating the medical system to provide a false diagnosis in the victim, but does not acknowledge any other aspects of MSbP.

Notably, neither sets of criteria are directed at clearly diagnosing an individual or a family. Instead, the focus lies on diagnosing a situation. Hence, attempts to develop diagnostic criteria that might appear in the International Classification of Diseases (ICD) system or the Diagnostic and Statistical Manual for Mental Disorders (DSM) have been challenging, because it is not clear "who" or "what" is carrying the resulting diagnosis. The current status is that the DSM-V includes diagnostic criteria for "factitious disorder imposed on another," the following of which all must be met for a positive diagnosis: (1) making up physical or psychological signs or symptoms or causing injury or disease in another person with the intention to deceive, (2) presenting another person to others as sick, injured, or having problems functioning, (3) continuing with the deception, even without receiving any visible benefit or reward, and (4) behavior is not better explained by another mental disorder [37]. Clearly, the aim is diagnosing the perpetrator of MSbP. However, the DSM does not define diagnostic criteria for victims of MSbP.

2.3. Challenges to studying MSbP victims

In the evolution of understanding this condition, the focus has been mainly on the perpetrators, and not the victims, even though the victims experience a high death rate, and many believe the perpetrators are untreatable [18, 38]. The study of child victims has been hampered by the general inability of systems designed to protect children from abuse, such as the medical system and child-protective systems, to successfully intervene to protect the victims [39–41].

In many identified cases of MSbP where unequivocal evidence of abuse exists, victims could not be successfully separated from perpetrators, and follow-up on the victims was not possible. For various reasons, including the fact that when cases were identified, the victims were found to already have dead siblings [42], it is believed that many identified victims went on to die or experience severe disability. Without follow-up, little is known about the actual mortality rate of victims, although case series studies of MSbP infant deaths originally misclassified as SIDS suggest that the mortality rate is high [1, 43–45]

Only one study exists of adult victims, an unscientific report of a case series of 10 surviving adults [46]. Although these adult victims "identified themselves as victims of childhood MSbP [and] volunteered to participate in research after learning of the author's work in this area through television or newspaper coverage," the author wrote about these patients with antipathy and incredulity: "Even before considering the question of how representative a sample this is, we are faced with the inevitable question of whether these subjects' stories are credible" [46]. Thus, this deeply flawed article represents the entirety of what is known about adult survivors of childhood MSbP.

2.4. Challenges to developing a patient-centered perspective on MSbP

The evolution of knowledge about MSbP in the scientific literature has been fractured for several reasons. First, inconsistent use of naming has challenged those who want to review all the literature on this topic, causing them to miss some literature because of this diversity of terms [47]. Next, a focus on understanding the perpetrator and perhaps treating him or her has intrigued psychologists, but has not produced any evidence-based course of action leading to a cure for these people [48]. This focus distracts from developing a public health approach to early identification and intervention, or even prevention, of this deadly child abuse.

This distraction includes perseverating over whether video surveillance of the perpetrator (resulting in the recording of MSbP abuse) is ethical or legal [49–52], as many cases reported in the literature could not have been identified using video surveillance due to the nature of the abuse. As one of many examples, Brink and Thackeray report on a 11-month-old infant repeatedly presenting to the emergency department (ED) after a foster mother consistently reported symptoms of a seizure disorder that could not be confirmed in a clinical setting [53].

Because much MSbP abuse cannot be recorded in a medical facility, such extended philosophical debate can be seen as a distraction from formulating practical public health recommendations aimed at early identification and prevention of MSbP.

2.5. Current lack of a patient-centered perspective on MSbP

Perhaps the most prominent obstacle to developing a patient-centered perspective on early intervention or prevention of MSbP has to do with the nature of the literature itself. It has only been tentatively acknowledged in the medical literature that while the perpetrator manipulates the medical system, it is actually the medical system's actions that ultimately are responsible for the injury and death experienced by MSbP victims [54–56]. Hence, the medical system is not held accountable for its contribution to MSbP morbidity and mortality.

While individual clinicians have sought to try to approach MSbP from a more public health- and patient-centered perspective [24, 25, 57, 58], their attempts are thwarted by the lack of a patient-centered perspective in the actual case reports and case series reports that are published in the scientific literature that provide the evidence base that informs them. Most case reports, from the history of reporting on this condition to the present time, focus on horrific medical details of the abuse, rather than the medical system's contribution to it [59–62]. For example, a 2015 report found that a mother was inserting real stones in her male child's urethra to try to convince clinicians that he had kidney stones; this child was returned to his family and no follow-up was done to see if the child was eventually killed [63]. It is common to see in these case reports that children are returned to the home of the perpetrator, even though there is no curative treatment for MSbP behavior, and the likelihood of the child's death is high [39]. Without follow-up, the actual mortality rate from MSbP abuse cannot be ascertained, and most case reports not only do not present follow-up information, but clearly do not even attempt it [39, 59–63].

This chapter represents a unique contribution to the MSbP literature in that it recommends a patient-centered perspective in the development of public health policy aimed at early identification and intervention, and possibly even prevention, of MSbP abuse. It provides practical, patient-centered recommendations that can be implemented as federal, state, and local healthcare policy with the focus of protecting the MSbP victim patient from the morbidity and mortality introduced by the medical system as part of MSbP.

3. The contributions of the healthcare system to MSbP morbidity and mortality

In order to develop a patient-centered perspective on prevention of and intervention on MSbP, it is important to first delineate how the healthcare system contributes to MSbP morbidity and mortality. This section reviews the literature that reports on case studies and case series of MSbP identified in a clinical setting and identifies in these cases what actions the healthcare system took that may have contributed to morbidity and mortality in MSbP victims.

This section starts by describing the healthcare system's contribution to MSbP abuse from a system perspective, not from an individual perspective. Next, this section reviews the evidence that certain providers within the healthcare system may actually carry a current diagnosis of "factitious disorder imposed on another," and discusses how the healthcare system may contribute to MSbP from an individual perspective.

3.1. How healthcare contributes to MSbP morbidity and mortality: system perspective

There are two principle ways in which the healthcare system contributes to morbidity and mortality in MSbP victims: (1) failure to take an action that is indicated by circumstances and (2) taking an action that would not be indicated had MSbP been identified. These contributions to MSbP morbidity and mortality can take place at various stages of treatment, including initial presentation, while attempting diagnosis, during treatment, and after MSbP is identified. This section describes failures of the healthcare system in early MSbP identification and intervention.

3.1.1. Not identifying MSbP at initial presentation

The primary contribution of the health-care system to MSbP at initial presentation is in failure to take an action indicated by circumstances. These include not properly investigating two main indications: indications of "doctor shopping" or multiple suspicious prior hospitalizations, and indications of MSbP symptoms in guardian gleaned from clinical interviews.

3.1.1.1. "Doctor shopping" and suspicious prior hospitalizations

Many MSbP cases present to clinical care with evidence of "doctor shopping" or multiple suspicious prior hospitalizations [62, 64–68]. Vadysinghe and Dayaratne describe a case in which "a three-year-old boy who has had repeated episodes of gross hematuria since the age of seven months" where no etiology could be found [68]. It was not until the child was age 3 that MSbP was even considered as a cause [68]. Green et al. describe diagnosing insulin poisoning in "an 8-week-old male infant with a history of multiple ED visits" without considering the multiple visits as possible indicators of child abuse [65].

Narang et al. report on a family of three children presenting at multiple hospitals over years with lesions on their faces of unknown etiology until the mother was identified as the MSbP perpetrator, burning their faces with a toilet cleaner [66]. In hindsight, the clinicians regret they did not consider MSbP earlier and list several sources of delay in diagnosis, including affirmative bias ("nobody suspects a parent would harm their child because the perpetrators appear as devoted parents"), the physician's pursuit of diagnosing a rare disease, unneeded medical interventions complicating the picture, and that children often are co-opted into the abuse dynamic and do not speak up [66]. Some of this delay in MSbP diagnosis could have been prevented if "doctor shopping" and multiple suspicious prior hospitalizations had been seen as potential indicators of MSbP behavior earlier in the course of diagnosis and treatment.

3.1.1.2. Failing to recognize MSbP symptoms in perpetrating guardian

Another healthcare system contribution to MSbP abuse at initial presentation is through failure to recognize MSbP symptoms in the perpetrating guardian from clinical interviews [42, 69]. In one case, clinicians failed to consider MSbP in a mother even after she lodged multiple fabricated accusations that neighbors and others were raping her son [69], though lodging false allegations of sexual abuse was identified as a potential indicator of MSbP behavior as early as 1996 [70].

At initial presentation, if the guardian becomes upset when diagnostic procedures are not initiated, this is also a potential indicator of MSbP behavior, which was missed in the case of the family of children whose faces were burned by a toilet cleaner [66]. Another potential indicator of MSbP behavior is multiple dead children in the family at initial presentation [42, 65, 71]. In a child victim of MSbP where the abuse was identified, the missed diagnosis of poisoning with sodium hydroxide, a household cleaner, led to the prior death of the child's sibling [72]. Another red flag apparent at initial presentation is the guardian speaking on behalf of the child in an inappropriate way. Dorothy Black described her interview with a woman suffering from Munchausen syndrome when "it was found that her three children were affected by proxy," and this was identified from a careful and thorough clinical interview [73].

There are many potential indicators of MSbP behavior at initial presentation revealed in case studies. Clinicians knew about these indicators, but did not realize their relationship to MSbP and therefore did not consider this etiology until much later in the course of diagnosis and treatment of the fabricated or induced illness. Lack of investigation into prior suspicious hospitalizations or multiple changes in care providers, and inability to recognize MSbP symptoms at initial presentation result in the healthcare system prolonging or completely missing that this type of child abuse is taking place, thus contributing substantially to the morbidity and mortality in MSbP victims.

3.1.2. Not identifying MSbP during the diagnostic stage

If MSbP abuse is not identified at initial presentation by the healthcare system, the patient can move to the next step, which is undergoing diagnostics by the healthcare system for the fabricated or induced illness. At this step, actual harm can be done by the healthcare system by subjecting the victims to unneeded invasive diagnostic procedures.

Although the healthcare system actively induces morbidity and mortality at the diagnostic step if victims are subjected to unnecessary diagnostic investigations and treatments, a more common healthcare system contribution to MSbP abuse at the diagnostic stage is failure to take indicated actions. One such action is ascertaining if the perpetrator (and even child victim) is lying; a second is by taking steps to observe specimen collection so it can be determined if specimens are being contaminated by the perpetrator. A third indicated action is to consider MSbP as a diagnosis and rule it out before proceeding, and a fourth indicated action is to take immediate action to protect the victim if MSbP is suspected. These contributions of the healthcare system to MSbP abuse will be further described here.

3.1.2.1. Initiation of invasive diagnostic procedures prompted by perpetrator's reports only

At the diagnostic step, the healthcare system can cause injury and illness by the initiation of invasive diagnostic procedures prompted only by perpetrator's report of symptoms with no clinical evidence of symptoms [62, 64, 68]. In a report about two teenage sisters who "presented with 2 years of gross hematuria and new onset heavy proteinuria," extensive diagnostic investigations are reported [62]. After finally considering MSbP, the clinicians found that the diagnoses of hematuria and proteinuria was due to the guardian's contamination of urine specimen and that "the children in our report are cases of child abuse in a medical setting (CAMS) due to exogenous added blood from unknown sources" [62].

The authors fail to recognize that their lack of identification of CAMS led to 2 years of trauma these sisters suffered at the hands of the healthcare system by subjecting them to extensive diagnostics on the basis of laboratory tests only. Had MSbP been considered early in the course of these diagnostics and the perpetrator identified, these sisters would have been protected from 2 years of this medical trauma.

3.1.2.2. Failing to ascertain if the perpetrator is lying

As the diagnostic stage, as at the initial presentation stage, the healthcare system more commonly contributes to MSbP abuse by not taking indicated actions. Ascertaining if the perpetrator is lying is possible at the diagnostic stage, since the healthcare system has more access to the perpetrator than at initial presentation. If the perpetrator is able to make it past the initial presentation into the diagnostic step, clinicians are afforded a chance to interview and observe the suspected guardian at length.

Unfortunately, action is often not taken due to lack of belief that perpetrators may be lying, or that a child may be co-opted into the fabrication [64, 74]. In a case where a mother was chronically poisoning her child with ipecac, producing a confusing clinical picture, clinicians simply believed her when "she denied any knowledge of environmental factors that could have caused these symptoms and denied any possibility of a toxic ingestion" [75]. Their failure to suspect the perpetrator led to a "hospital course … marked by complex clinical findings requiring several interventions" without any consideration of an MSbP diagnosis [75]. As with the article on fabricated gross hematuria in two sisters [62], the authors failed to recognize their contribution to the child's trauma at the hands of the medical system due to the inaction of members of the system.

Shapiro and Nguyen point out that clinicians must consider that not only the perpetrator but also the child victim may be lying, as he or she may have been co-opted into the abuse dynamic [74]. These authors describe a teenage boy who "was medically knowledgeable and could recount with great detail his supposed multiple medical conditions and symptoms" while continuing to endorse "symptoms of his reported medical illnesses of which there were no objective signs" [74].

This phenomenon is understandable, considering that the perpetrator is usually the mother and has cultivated a mother-child relationship without boundaries and where the child has been coached and offered positive reinforcement of their relationship only from cooperating with the abuse. This phenomenon was demonstrated in the young adult child of a mother engaging in MSbP abuse [76]. When clinicians "found a syringe containing cloudy fluid with an uncapped needle underneath [the patient] in her bed," it was soon determined that this needle must have come from the mother, because the hospital did not use that type of needle [76]. When this was discussed in front of the patient and the mother, the mother insisted the syringe was the patient's, and the patient never spoke at all [76]. The patient was discharged and 2 weeks later died of sepsis secondary to being injected with a fluid contaminated with what was believed to be "ear wax" [76]. In this case, the healthcare system contributed directly to the victim's death by not considering that the adult child and her mother were lying.

3.1.2.3. Failure to directly observe specimen collection

Several cases point to contamination of specimens at the diagnostic stage as reasons that clinicians proceed to the treatment stage, falsely believing the evidence indicated a legitimate diagnosis. In the case of the 3-year-old boy treated for repeated episodes of gross hematuria since he was 7 months old, clinicians finally began to suspect the mother as a perpetrator after they found that "urine which was collected under supervision showed no gross hematuria, while the urine which was collected by the mother was red in color" [68]. Likewise, in the teenage sisters who were treated for 2 years for hematuria and proteinuria, "collect[ing] clean-catch urine under direct staff supervision was refused" by the perpetrator, thus delaying the diagnosis of MSbP [62]. Analysis resulted in the findings that the urine contained "body fluids or tissue from more than one individual," finally prompting clinicians to conclude that the perpetrator had been tampering with the specimens [62].

Repeated contradictory laboratory findings, which are also contradicted by clinical signs and symptoms, should encourage clinicians to rule out MSbP abuse. This can be done by observing the specimen collection. Refusal of the guardian to allow observed specimen collection is itself an indication of MSbP. By not being aware of this information, clinicians may not take action to rule out MSbP and thus induce the healthcare system to contribute to the morbidity and mortality of MSbP victims.

3.1.2.4. Failing to consider MSbP as a differential diagnosis when indicated

A third way the healthcare system can fail to act during the diagnostic stage is by simply failing to consider a differential diagnosis of MSbP as a possible cause for confusing, poorly established, or contradictory evidence of a diagnosis [67]. As Criddle describes in her overview of MSbP, the old healthcare maxim, "When you hear hoofbeats, think horses, not zebras" suggests that the first step in clarifying a confusing diagnostic picture in children should not be the consideration of a rare disease, but rather the consideration that some of the diagnostic information has been manipulated [77].

This lack of consideration of MSbP is seen in the healthcare system's hot pursuit of rare medical diagnoses at the diagnostic stage, which technically should be put off until an MSbP diagnosis is ruled out. In fact, a clinician named Steinschneider in 1972 failed to consider murder as a possible cause of serial deaths in multiple children in a family due to suffocation by an MSbP mother, while Steinschneider pursued explanation of their deaths by some other etiology [78]. Steinschneider eventually published a paper advocating that the children died of a mysterious "sudden infant death syndrome," thus establishing SIDS as a possible diagnosis [78], which later led to many MSbP perpetrators escaping prosecution after murdering their children [1, 43, 79], as well as a 1996 retraction of Steinschneider's original article [7].

As data-driven example, the prevalence rate of MSbP has been estimated in a few countries. McClure and colleagues estimated that "the combined annual incidence of these conditions in children aged under 16 years is at least 0.5 per 100,000 and for children aged under 1, at least 2.81 per 100,000" in the United Kingdom (UK) [71]. Denny et al. reported "the incidence rate for MSBP in children aged less than 16 years was 2.0 per 100,000 children" in New Zealand [80].

Compare this to the consideration of a diagnosis of Rabson-Mendenhall syndrome, which was described in one case study of MSbP abuse [67]. The NORD Guide to Rare Disorders indicates that Rabson-Mendenhall syndrome is a result of an inherited autosomal-recessive trait and says the prevalence of this syndrome is "believed to be approximately 1 in 1 million" [81]. Another case study of MSbP abuse described considering a diagnosis of Gaucher disease [82]. The NORD Guide to Rare Disorders does not estimate the incidence of this disease, only to point out that the highest prevalence is in Ashkenazic Jews (one in 800 births) and that there were only 7500 Gaucher disease patients in the US as of the book's writing [81]. Another report describes considering cicatricial pemphigoid as the diagnosis in what turned out to be MSbP abuse where the perpetrator was giving a child oral sodium hydroxide, a household cleaning product [72]. The NORD guide does report a higher prevalence of this condition at one in 12,000 to one in 20,000, but notes that "the disease most often occurs in patients 60 years of age or older," not children [81].

Although rates of MSbP in only the UK and New Zealand have been reported, it is generally believed that rates are higher, mainly due to the suspected undercounting of cases when the identification of known cases reveals that there are existing dead siblings in the family [71]. The youngest children are at a highest risk [71], so ruling out MSbP early should be an action taken by the healthcare system prior to investigations into rarer diseases.

The healthcare system can also miss overt presentations of MSbP that go unnoticed by clinicians simply because of their lack of knowledge of the condition. For example, poisonings are common presentations of MSbP. A review of 87 case studies reporting MSbP poisonings reveals a time trend associated with the mechanism used in poisoning (see **Figure 1**).

As can be seen from the figure, prior to 1984, the mechanism of poisoning in MSbP was more likely to be tranquilizers and antidepressants, while between 1985 and 1999, emetics, chiefly ipecac, was a mechanism used commonly in MSbP poisonings. Ipecac was originally recommended by poison control centers as an approach to controlling accidental poisonings in children; other approaches were more strongly recommended as of 2004 and the availability of ipecac declined such that this trend in MSbP poisoning became less prevalent [147]. Starting in 2000, insulin became a more common mechanism behind MSbP poisoning.

http://dx.doi.org/10.5772/65814

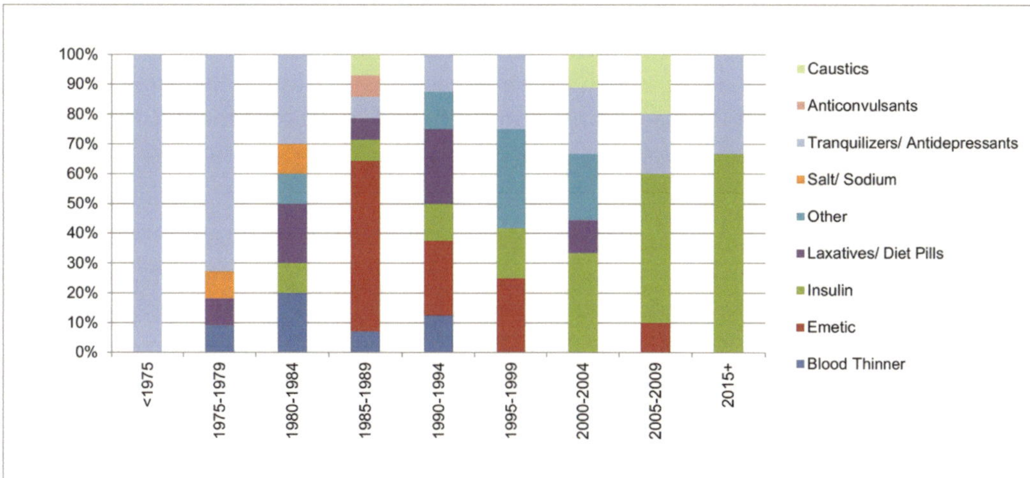

Figure 1. Distribution of mechanisms of MSbP poisonings in peer-reviewed case studies, 1965–2015. Case study Refs.: [9, 12, 20, 21, 31, 41, 42, 46, 47, 60, 65, 67, 72, 75, 83–146]. Please note that some of these articles present multiple case reports, and the figure reflects counts of case reports, not articles. "Other" includes lye, pepper, rat poison, frusemide (diuretic), arsenic, caffeine, antihistamines, clonidine (blood pressure medication), opioids, lead, mercury, and tetrahydrozoline (eye drops).

This lack of knowledge about common MSbP presentations, such as poisonings, is an important way that healthcare systems contribute to MSbP abuse at the diagnostic stage [42, 60, 65, 135]. Failure of clinicians to recognize salt [135] and insulin poisoning [42, 60, 65], as well as perpetrator-induced septicemia or polymicrobial bacteremia [82, 148], can lead victims to experience more MSbP-abuse-related morbidity and mortality as they suffer from the abuse by the perpetrator, while advancing to later stages of treatment for a fictitious or induced condition, thus suffering abuse from the healthcare system itself.

3.1.2.5. Failure to act upon suspicion of MSbP abuse

A fourth way the healthcare system contributes to MSbP abuse is its failure to act immediately upon suspicion of MSbP abuse [60, 149]. In their case study of a child who was repeatedly insulin-poisoned, Loo and Yap appear to not realize that the ingestion of insulin was not accidental [60]. In the Kathy Bush case, detailed later in this chapter, most clinicians felt that the mother involved was an MSbP perpetrator, and there was much evidence of MSbP abuse, including confirmed tampering with specimens [150]. Even so, the healthcare system colluded with the mother to perpetrate 8 years of severe MSbP abuse of Mrs. Bush's daughter [150].

With amazing insight, Yalndağ-Öztürk and colleagues explain in their article that "failure to properly diagnose MSbP can lead to further abuse by the caregiver and increase the risk of complications due to long hospital stays and invasive tests. In this paper, we describe our experiences with a baby who ended up being diagnosed with MSbP, including our initial failure to find a pathology, delay of MSbP diagnosis, our growing suspicion of MSbP despite technical setbacks, our actions after we confirmed MSbP as the cause of his hospitalizations" [149]. This demonstrates that even if a clinician is trained in common MSbP presentations, yet he or she fails to act upon suspicion of an MSbP case immediately at the diagnostic stage, there can be prolonged MSbP abuse of the victim, with additional contribution of the healthcare system to this abuse by prolonging diagnosis and treatment of a fictitious or induced condition in the victim.

3.1.3. Not identifying MSbP abuse during the treatment stage

A particularly damaging way the healthcare system contributes to MSbP abuse at the treatment stage is by initiating treatment or procedures despite confusing, poorly established, or contradictory evidence of a diagnosis. However, the healthcare system also can contribute to MSbP abuse at the treatment stage by simply failing to consider MSbP when the treatments do not work, and by failing to recognize hostility in the victim's guardian when stopping medical treatment, two indications that MSbP abuse should be ruled out immediately.

3.1.3.1. Initiating treatment for a poorly established diagnosis

The healthcare system can contribute heavily to the MSbP abuse suffered by victims by the provision of treatment or initiation of procedures in the face of confusing, poorly established, or contradictory evidence of a diagnosis [143, 151]. Perhaps the most famous case of the healthcare system contributing heavily to the abuse of an MSbP victim was that of Kathy Bush. Mrs. Bush, who was convicted by a jury in Florida of child abuse, was found to have over the course of 8 years "repeatedly, directly, or through physicians attempting to diagnose and treat non-existent conditions, caused her [daughter] grave bodily harm (e.g., some 40 operations)" [150].

While Mrs. Bush was convicted, no one in the healthcare system involved in any of these 40 operations was held accountable for the healthcare system's failure to protect the child. Although MSbP abuse was suspected since the child was 3 years of age, it was not stopped until 8 years later [150], directly implicating the healthcare system with failure to protect the child from these unneeded treatments.

In his article on the case, Schreier points out that 21 of the 22 nurses treating the child felt that her mother was an MSbP perpetrator, the mother was found to have been contaminating specimens, and the mother became so hostile as to actually file a lawsuit against the hospital when they sent material to a laboratory for investigation into potential MSbP abuse without her permission or a doctor's order [150]. The child had been subjected to multiple feeding tubes, and as part of the court trial, the gastroenterologist at the center treating the child admitted that "there had never been any need for these surgically implanted feeding tubes" [150].

Even under these conditions of grave medical malpractice, resulting in serious harm to the child, no one in the healthcare system was held accountable. In his article, Schreier does not address this point and seems to blame the perpetrator entirely for the abuse that was ultimately delivered repeatedly to the victim by the healthcare system, despite many actors in the system knowing that these treatments were constituting abuse.

This fact is startling to reflect upon when considering the multiple licensure procedures, regulations, and accreditations healthcare facilities must undergo in the US, coupled with the high levels of sophistication in the medical system participants in the abuse, compared to the relative unsophistication of an MSbP perpetrator. At one point, the perpetrator even appealed for financial help, citing a lack of resources to continue to pay for treatments [150]. Ironically, many children with real chronic diseases go without necessary treatment in the US due to lack of funds; however, in the case of Kathy Bush, the healthcare system continued to contribute enthusiastically to the child's abuse, even when resources were running out [150].

Providing treatment for fabricated or induced illnesses might be the single most damaging action the healthcare system can take in contributing to MSbP abuse. For this reason, MSbP abuse that is not caught before the treatment stage can lead to a high level of participation by the healthcare system in the abuse MSbP victims experience at the treatment stage.

3.1.3.2. Failure to consider MSbP when treatments do not work

If MSbP abuse is not detected at initial presentation or the diagnostic stage and therefore proceeds to the treatment stage, MSbP needs to be considered when treatments do not work [42, 65, 66, 151]. In a case by Wagner and Bowers, a child with ongoing tachycardia was treated with no resolution, but during this treatment, MSbP was not considered as a potential cause [75]. During the treatment of several children in a family who were being insulin-poisoned by their mother, no clinicians suspected that the treatment was not working due to sabotage by the mother, thus resulting in multiple child deaths [42].

Diagnoses of falsified or induced illnesses are typically confusing and tentative, and this situation coupled with the repeated delivery of failed treatments should strongly suggest a need to rule out MSbP. It is particularly important for the healthcare system to step up and take accountability at the treatment stage, when most of the damage is done by the healthcare system to MSbP victims.

3.1.3.3. Failure to recognize hostility in guardian when stopping medical treatment

Because MSbP victims at the treatment stage are being treated for falsified or induced illness, it is at this stage that it may become apparent that the treatments are not indicated and should be removed. At that point, if the guardian becomes hostile, it is a clear indication that MSbP should be investigated. In a case of a mother inducing thigh abscesses in her daughter, "when discharge was discussed, the mother became hostile and started to blame medical personnel for her daughter's condition" [151]. In a case where a father and uncle were confronted after being found to be inducing emesis through poisoning of a child using betadine, the two "displayed anger and disbelief and insisted that their son should be immediately discharged and refused to contact the social services" [64]. In two other cases, parents refused to approve an autopsy after their baby died [42, 72].

These are clear indicators during the treatment stage that MSbP is a likely cause of the illness for which the child is being treated. When the healthcare system does not recognize these clear signs of MSbP perpetration, it becomes an accomplice MSbP perpetrator itself.

3.1.4. Contribution of the healthcare system to MSbP abuse after identification

MSbP abuse can be identified at the initial presentation stage, the diagnostic stage, and the treatment stage. Regardless of when the abuse is identified, the healthcare system has the responsibility of protecting the identified victim or victims and ensuring that follow-up occurs to mitigate their physical and psychological morbidity.

While the most likely contribution by the healthcare system to inducing mortality and morbidity in MSbP victims is unnecessary treatment, the most serious is lack of follow-up and treatment after MSbP is identified. This inaction can be characterized as not ensuring the victim's ongoing protection and not providing treatment for the physical and psychological comorbidity associated with the abuse suffered by the victim at the hands of the healthcare system. In fact, the healthcare system may take action to reunite the victim with the perpetrator, thus increasing the victim's risk. Actors within the healthcare system may also take steps to cover up its role in the abuse. Abuse at the hands of the healthcare system is the responsibility of the healthcare system.

3.1.4.1. Lack of ensuring victim protection

The Kathy Bush case illustrates a particularly stark example of lack of the healthcare system's accountability in accepting responsibility for protecting the identified victim once MSbP evidence was established, including lack of protection and follow-up with the victim, but there are many other examples of this failure of the healthcare system in the literature [63, 65, 68, 69, 150–154]. While many reports talk about separating the child from the perpetrator, such as having the child live with his or her father when the mother is found to be the perpetrator, safety is not insured because the perpetrator may still have access to victim [63, 64, 151, 154, 155]. In an article that contends that the "system worked", saying, "both [abused] children were removed out-of-state to their father's family" [155] away from the maternal abuser, the article fails to admit that this action does not actually ensure the ongoing safety of the victims. Having the abuser processed through the judicial system for child endangerment on the basis of the evidence gathered by the healthcare system will likely result in the removal of the abuser from society at large and only then will the victims actually be safe.

Because MSbP abuse is essentially attempted murder, there should be little difficulty in having the perpetrator detained by law enforcement once hard evidence of abuse is available. This evidence is only available through the healthcare system, which is the weapon being used in the attempted murder. Therefore, this evidence should be supplied to law enforcement so that charges of attempted murder can be brought against the perpetrator. A modern case where MSbP behavior by the mother, Lacey Spears, resulted in the death of her son, Garnett, was described this way: "To this day it's not clear how Lacey Spears, 27, convinced an Alabama surgeon to insert a gastric feeding tube into her son's stomach before he was a year old, after doctors at another hospital refused, saying it wasn't needed. What is now clear is this: Spears used the plastic tube as a murder weapon [156]." The "astonishing 23 trips to the hospital by Garnett's first birthday" should have tipped off the healthcare system [156]. Had healthcare played a role in supplying evidence to law enforcement, rather than avoiding the perpetrator or being coerced into participating in the crime, Garnett's life may have been saved. Because many MSbP perpetrators have multiple victims, an easy case can be made for the danger of the perpetrator to society, and detention or constant observation of the perpetrator is required to maintain the safety of the identified victim or victims, should they still be alive.

Many authors of case studies complain of the difficulty of working with child-protective services and other agencies to ensure the victim's safety. Kathryn Artingstall provides useful guidance in her book, "Practical Aspects of Munchausen by Proxy and Munchausen Syndrome Investigation" [157]. Much of the challenge lies in gathering the evidence of abuse; once this is available, charging the abuser with attempted murder is much less difficult [157].

3.1.4.2. Lack of ensuring rehabilitative care

Victims of MSbP abuse, like other victims of torture, require extensive rehabilitative treatment after being removed from the abuse situation. A discussion of the healthcare system's responsibility in providing this treatment once MSbP abuse is identified is almost completely absent from the scientific literature [63, 65, 68, 69, 152–154]. One article reports that "the patient was discharged after being scheduled for control visits at related departments," which is unclear and suggests that follow-up rehabilitative treatment was not ensured [153]. In another case, where an MSbP perpetrator was orally administering household cleaner causing lesions on the victim, the article only discusses that the lesions that appearing as a result of the poisoning resolved, but makes no mention of treatment for victimization [72].

The healthcare system's lack in providing appropriate rehabilitative care to identified MSbP victims is somewhat astonishing. Once chronic ipecac poisoning was identified in a case study of MSbP abuse, the authors concluded, "This child [victim] was from a neighboring state, making the jurisdiction for both criminal and social service involvement complicated. After much discussion between both states, the patient was transferred to a tertiary care center in his home state for resolution of criminal and social work issues and determination of appropriate discharge placement" [75]. In the article that contended the "system worked," the healthcare system did not ensure that the children removed from the home were treated for child abuse [155].

This lack of rehabilitative services is particularly counterintuitive, since the healthcare system is designed to provide these services. On the other hand, the healthcare system is not designed to provide health care for fabricated or induced illness. Yet, the healthcare system participates at high levels in delivering the abuse, then seems to "wash its hands" of the victims as soon as the abuse is identified. Instead of delivering needed care to the victims of MSbP abuse to aid in healing the abuse, it only participates in delivering unneeded care in the form of abuse.

3.2. How health care contributes to MSbP morbidity and mortality: individual perspective

The previous section discussed how the healthcare system contributes to morbidity and mortality in MSbP victims. Unfortunately, individual healthcare providers themselves can be direct MSbP abusers. A few examples where providers were confirmed to be MSbP perpetrators exist in the literature, and these will be reviewed. Next, cases in the lay press that appear to be examples of MSbP provider perpetrators who have not been specifically investigated for MSbP abuse will be examined. Finally, how the troubled teen industry (TTI) serves as an attractive setting for MSbP perpetrators will be discussed.

3.2.1. Confirmed MSbP perpetrators who were healthcare providers

In one article, an MSbP perpetrator is described as a nurse who administered benzodiazepines, morphine, and other drugs to infants [86]. When the infants became intoxicated, she sought help for the babies and comforted the family in the face of the situation's uncertainty [86]. Eventually, the nurse was convicted and served time in jail [86].

In another case study of a provider who was an MSbP perpetrator, a nursing student, "Judy", was found to be poisoning an infant with laxatives and preventing discharge of her child victims. "Ironically, although Judy was charged with child abuse, she continued in the second year of the nursing program. Faculty were unaware of the charge and Judy knew that they would not be informed under privacy legislation" [144], so in this case, the healthcare system did not protect its patients from a known perpetrator on their staff.

3.2.2. Unconfirmed MSbP perpetrators who were healthcare providers

Other cases of providers abusing patients have been identified, but have not been determined to be MSbP due to lack of investigation into the potential MSbP aspects of the abuse. In the book, "The Good Nurse: A True Story of Medicine, Madness, and Murder," author Charles Graeber describes a true story about how nurse Charles Cullen may have killed up to 400 intensive care unit (ICU) patients by injecting them with high levels of digoxin, a heart medication [158]. No motive was identified for these murders, and MSbP as a motive was not investigated [158]. Cullen's killing went unchecked because when the deaths were suspected to be murders by one hospital, its administrators would quietly prompt Cullen to resign, saying they would provide a letter of recommendation for his employment at a subsequent hospital if he resigned, in an effort to avoid a lawsuit against the hospital [158]. Eventually, Cullen confessed to some of the murders, and was convicted [158].

Another recent case of a healthcare provider potentially being an MSbP perpetrator is in the case of Justina Pelletier, a teenager from Connecticut who was being treated in Massachusetts for mitochondrial disorder, a rare and poorly understood condition [159]. When she was being transferred from one Boston hospital to Boston Children's for care based on a referral, she was virtually kidnapped by Boston Children's healthcare providers and locked in the psychiatric unit, where they withdrew her medications, thus causing her health to deteriorate [159]. Further, child-protective services were called to investigate the parents, who showed no signs or symptoms of being MSbP abusers [159]. However, involving child-protective services for false accusations of abuse is itself a symptom of MSbP perpetration [160]. These actions were indications that the individual orchestrating this abuse was indeed a provider at Children's Hospital.

The provider behind the actions at Boston Children's that kept Pelletier wrongly imprisoned for 18 months, according to her family, was identified as Dr. Alice Newton in a lawsuit filed by the Pelletier family in 2016 [161]. Dr. Newton had already been profiled in the Boston Globe, which noted that, "In the past few years, [Newton's] medical judgment has been openly questioned in three high-profile cases, two of which involved shaken-baby abuse charges that were later dropped" [162].

http://dx.doi.org/10.5772/65814

Eerie parallels can be drawn between the case of Dr. Newton and the career arc of Dr. Meadow, the British pediatrician who originally named MSbP in 1976, as described in the first section of this chapter. Dr. Meadow later went on to be accused of falsely convicting innocent parents of being MSbP abusers. In the particularly high-profile case of Sally Clark, Meadow had her jailed for MSbP when her infant died; she was later released when it was determined that the child actually succumbed to meningitis [163]. Clark died shortly after being released from jail, having never recovered from the dual trauma of losing her baby and being falsely convicted of MSbP abuse at the hands of Meadow [163].

As explained by clinician James LeFanu in a letter to the Lancet, "Meadow's contention that two or more unexplained deaths in the same family is murder until proved otherwise (commonly known as 'Meadow's Rule') was based on his own experience, not rigorous statistics, and this is part of what led to the successful conviction of many innocent parents and guardians who he falsely accused of MSbP abuse" [164]. LeFanu explained how it happened this way: "Thus, the façade of expertise on the potentially sinister cause of recurrent infant death that Meadow presented to the court proves on close examination to be built on insecure foundations, although regrettably juries, for a time, found it sufficiently persuasive to cause them to compound the unimaginable suffering of bereaved mothers with a life sentence" [164].

Meadow, though knighted for his supposed contribution to the protection of MSbP-abused children, was scolded in a letter from the President of the Royal Statistical Society for making up statistics that greatly overstated the likelihood that MSbP was responsible for child deaths in several cases [165]. In addition to the Clark case, four other cases that Meadow provided expert witness in convicting were overturned [163]. Sally Clark's father eventually brought Meadow to the General Medical Council where he was found guilty of "serious professional misconduct" [166].

3.2.3. The troubled teen industry

In his book, "Institutionalized Persuasion," Marcus Chatfield reviews how unregulated healthcare settings in the troubled teen industry (TTI), such as S.A.F.E. and S.T.R.A.I.G.H.T., may actually serve as magnets for MSbP provider abusers, the way daycare settings are an attraction for pedophiles [167]. These facilities essentially convince parents to give up their teenage children into an institutionalized setting under the guise of substance-abuse treatment, only to subject them to MSbP-like abuse by providing unstudied "treatments" that are akin to brainwashing and prisoner-of-war torture [167]. Though these healthcare settings have been cited for causing serious injury and death in the children who participate, there is no federal regulation against their existence, so even when a facility is found to be guilty of criminal behavior and is closed, other ones quickly open [167]. The mere existence of the TTI is evidence that MSbP provider perpetrators exist and can easily play into the hands of MSbP guardian perpetrators who are seeking providers to deliver unneeded care for fabricated or induced illnesses.

The mere existence of TTI pushes the question: What qualifies as a "healthcare setting"? An ED seems to be a healthcare setting, but an ED that refuses to treat pain is essentially a torture chamber, as it is not upholding its ethical duty to relieve pain and suffering [168]. The realization that physicians in World War II acted as torturers under the guise of "medical research" led to our modern day ethical boards to protect human subjects in research. This suggests that simply having people we call "healthcare practitioners" acting in something we casually call a "healthcare setting" does not necessarily qualify it as a healthcare setting. In the case of TTI, "healthcare" is not being delivered. No evidence-based treatment for a particular condition is being administered by qualified practitioners.

This situation suggests that more regulation is needed on what is legally defined as a healthcare setting, and this would be necessary on the federal level to prevent TTI and other pseudo-healthcare settings from "state-shopping." This regulation is not only to prevent pseudo-healthcare setting such as the TTI from being maintained but also to prevent drift of traditional healthcare settings, such as an ED, into the area of disqualification due to lack of ethical conduct, by, for example, not adequately treating pain.

4. A patient-centered approach to preventing MSbP in the healthcare system

This section applies the Haddon matrix framework to develop recommendations on how to prevent or mitigate the healthcare system's contribution to MSbP abuse from both a functional perspective on the healthcare system as well as individuals employed in the healthcare system. The Haddon matrix was invented by William Haddon, Jr., and was originally intended as a framework "applying basic principles of public health to the problem of traffic safety" [169]. Per Haddon's original 1980 work, "A logical system for preventing injury and death in motor vehicle crashes is based on the sequence of events (pre-crash, crash, and post-crash) and types of factors involved (human, vehicle and equipment, physical environment and roadway, and socioeconomic environment)" [170]. He felt that creating a table, or a matrix, with the sequence of events along the rows and the types of factors in the columns, and then filling in the cells at the intersections, would represent a reasonable and systematic approach to weigh the various prevention and intervention options, and to evaluate the individual effectiveness of each proposed option [170].

Since its inception, it has been used as a framework for considering approaches to injury prevention in public health and has been used specifically for considering prevention of childhood injuries [171, 172]. In her 1998 paper, Carol Runyan provides examples of applying the Haddon matrix to prevent childhood injury [169]; the application of the Haddon matrix to the prevention and early intervention of MSbP abuse in the healthcare system will be delineated here.

The Haddon matrix encourages consideration of actions that can be taken pre-event, or before the healthcare system participates in MSbP abuse, during the event of the healthcare system participating in MSbP abuse, and post-event, after MSbP abuse is identified in the healthcare system. It considers the host, which is the healthcare system, the agent, which are unnecessary medical procedures, the physical environment, which is the healthcare setting, and the social environment, which are healthcare-related norms, policies, and rules.

As described in **Table 1**, much can be achieved through policymaking at both the federal and local levels. Federal regulation of the TTI can prevent MSbP abuse by providers in that setting, while state regulation can hold healthcare facilities accountable for having established protocols for intervening on identified MSbP cases as well as holding healthcare providers accountable for

http://dx.doi.org/10.5772/65814

Timing	*Host* – Healthcare System	*Agent/Vehicle* – Unnecessary Medical Procedures	*Physical Environment* – Clinical or Hospital Setting	*Social Environment* – Healthcare Norms, Policies and Rules
Pre-event – before healthcare system involvement in MSbP abuse	Regularly training pediatric providers to identify signs and symptoms of MSbP perpetration Before proceeding with diagnostic procedures, investigating when patient has had prior suspicious hospitalizations, or has presented at multiple facilities with the same complaint Training clinicians to recognize hostility in guardians in reaction to not proceeding with diagnostics as a sign of potential MSbP abuse	Prevention of invasive diagnostics based only on reports and not clinical observation Taking steps to confirm that guardians reporting signs and symptoms are not lying Ruling out MSbP abuse when indicated at initial presentation before proceeding with diagnostics, especially for a rare disease	Directly observing specimen collection Requiring immediate intervention by health-care providers on the suspicion of MSbP abuse	Screening of healthcare professionals for MSbP behavior prior to employment Providing protocol to follow when healthcare professionals identify non-provider MSbP abuse perpetrator Providing protocol to follow when healthcare professionals identify provider MSbP abuse perpetrator Enacting federal regulation of the Troubled Teen Industry (TTI)
Event – during healthcare system involvement in MSbP abuse	Ruling out MSbP early in the course of diagnosis or treatment as soon as signs or symptoms of MSbP are perceived	Not initiating invasive treatments before a legitimate diagnosis has been confirmed and MSbP has been ruled out When treatments are found not to work, immediately removing them and working to rule out MSbP abuse	Requiring immediate intervention by healthcare providers on the suspicion of MSbP abuse Recognizing the hostility of guardians to discontinuation of treatment as a sign of potential MSbP abuse	Providing support to intervening providers working through MSbP abuse identification protocols Immediately removing and convicting providers found to be engaging in MSbP abuse of their patients
Post-event – after identifying MSbP abuse in the heath-care system	Holding the healthcare system accountable for ensuring ongoing safety of identified victims Holding healthcare system accountable for providing comprehensive rehabilitative treatment to victims	Prevention of "doctor shopping" or the use of another component of the healthcare system by MSbP abuser for perpetration Prevention of provider MSbP abusers from working in a healthcare setting	After MSbP cases are identified, determining and implementing features to improve the healthcare setting so as to prevent further cases Using past experience to improve the early detection of MSbP cases	Holding healthcare professionals accountable for not intervening on known MSbP abuse Holding healthcare professionals accountable for knowingly participating in MSbP abuse

This table shows the results of Haddon's matrix applied to the issue of MSbP in the healthcare system.

Table 1. Haddon matrix applied to the problem of the healthcare system's contribution to MSbP.

proceeding through these protocols when indicated, thus ensuring victim safety after abuse is identified. State regulations can also hold healthcare facilities accountable for providing necessary follow-up treatment for victims. State regulation that holds healthcare facilities accountable for deliberately participating in MSbP abuse, either by not intervening when it is identified or by hiring providers who are MSbP perpetrators, will encourage healthcare settings to develop policies to screen out providers who are MSbP perpetrators, and to promote the immediate identification and early intervention on suspected MSbP cases. Healthcare settings can also create policy to indicate when directly observed specimen collection is needed.

Also shown in **Table 1** is that much can be achieved in the detection and early intervention of MSbP abuse through provider education. Clinicians, especially those who deal regularly with children such as pediatricians, can be fully educated on all the signs and symptoms of MSbP abuse, both when perpetrated by a guardian and when perpetrated by another healthcare provider. Regularly refreshing clinician knowledge of MSbP with updated information can go a long way toward helping clinicians identify immediately when MSbP abuse needs to be ruled out before diagnostic and treatment activities proceed.

5. Conclusion

In conclusion, although MSbP abuse results in severe morbidity and mortality in its victims, much can be done at the federal, state, and local levels to facilitate prevention and early intervention by focusing on the healthcare system's contribution to the abuse. This chapter first described the evolution of thought and understanding about MSbP abuse, and why the current literature lacks recommendations on patient-centered approaches to addressing this condition. The second section of this chapter reviewed how the healthare system contributes to MSbP abuse from both a system and individual perspective, and the third section of this chapter uses the Haddon matrix to present a patient-centered, public health framework to guide prevention and early intervention of MSbP abuse in the healthcare setting.

The authors hope that the presentation of information in this format will facilitate a greater understanding of the healthcare system's contribution to MSbP abuse, as well as promote holding the healthcare system accountable for its role in the abuse. We hope that the development of a public health, patient-centered framework for mitigating or possibly eliminating the MSbP abuse contributed by the healthcare system will lead to the healthcare system taking greater responsibility for its role in the abuse, and to leaders taking to take a greater responsibility for holding the healthcare system accountable.

Author details

Monika M. Wahi[1, 2]*, Kenton V. Stone[3], Mariel Chance[2] and Cynthia E. Miller[2]

*Address all correspondence to: mwahi@vasantahealth.com

1 Laboure College, Milton, MA, USA

2 Vasanta Health Science, Cambridge, MA, USA

3 Allegany College of Maryland, Cumberland, MD, USA

http://dx.doi.org/10.5772/65814

References

[1] Craft AW, Hall DMB. Munchausen syndrome by proxy and sudden infant death. Br Med J 2004;328:1309–12. doi:10.1136/bmj.328.7451.1309.

[2] Liebrechts-Akkerman G, Lao O, Liu F, van Sleuwen BE, Engelberts AC, L'Hoir MP, et al. Postnatal parental smoking: an important risk factor for SIDS. Eur J Pediatr 2011;170:1281–91. doi:10.1007/s00431-011-1433-6.

[3] Centers for Disease Control and Prevention. Sudden Infant Death Syndrome (SIDS) and Sudden, Unexpected Infant Death (SUID) – Reproductive Health. Cent Dis Control Prev 2016. https://www.cdc.gov/sids/(accessed August 6, 2016).

[4] Becroft DM, Lockett BK. SIDS or murder? Pediatrics 1998;101:953–5.

[5] Emery JL, Chandra S, Gilbert-Barness EF. Findings in child deaths registered as sudden infant death syndrome (SIDS) in Madison, Wisconsin. Pediatr Pathol 1988;8:171–8.

[6] Geelhoed GC, Pemberton PJ. SIDS, seizures or 'esophageal reflux? Another manifestation of Munchausen syndrome by proxy. Med J Aust 1985;143:357–8.

[7] Steinschneider A. Prolonged apnea and the sudden infant death syndrome: clinical and laboratory observations. Pediatrics 1994;93:944.

[8] Meadow R. Munchausen syndrome by proxy: the hinterland of child abuse. The Lancet 1977:343–5.

[9] Osborne JP. Non-accidental poisoning and child abuse. Br Med J 1976;1:1211.

[10] Birrell RG, Birrell JH. The maltreatment syndrome in children: a hospital survey. Med J Aust 1968;2:1023–9.

[11] Hodge III D, Schwartz W, Sargent J, Bodurtha J, Starr S. The bacteriologically battered baby: another case of Munchausen by proxy. Ann Emerg Med 1982;11:205–7. doi:10.1016/S0196-0644(82)80499-X.

[12] Shnaps Y, Frand M, Rotem Y, Tirosh M. The chemically abused child. Pediatrics 1981;68:119–21.

[13] Bass C, Jones D. Psychopathology of perpetrators of fabricated or induced illness in children: case series. Br J Psychiatry J Ment Sci 2011;199:113–8. doi:10.1192/bjp.bp.109.074088.

[14] Bools C, Neale B, Meadow R. Munchausen syndrome by proxy: a study of psychopathology. Child Abuse Negl 1994;18:773–88.

[15] Libow JA, Schreier HA. Three forms of factitious illness in children: when is it Munchausen syndrome by proxy? Am J Orthopsychiatry 1986;56:602–11.

[16] Ackerman NB Jr, Strobel CT. Polle syndrome: chronic diarrhea in Munchausen's child. Gastroenterology 1981;81:1140–2.

[17] Casavant MJ. Polle's syndrome (Munchausen by proxy). Pediatr Emerg Care 1995;11:264.

[18] Adshead G, Bluglass K. A vicious circle: transgenerational attachment representations in a case of factitious illness by proxy. Attach Hum Dev 2001;3:77–95. doi:10.1080/14616730010024780.

[19] Ahmed ZE. Factitious disorder imposed on another (Munchausen syndrome by proxy), a potentially lethal form of child abuse. J Child Adolesc Behav 2015;3. doi:10.4172/2375-4494.1000e106:e106.

[20] Arnold SM, Arnholz D, Garyfallou GT, Heard K. Two siblings poisoned with diphenhydramine: a case of factitious disorder by proxy. Ann Emerg Med 1998;32:256–9. doi:10.1016/S0196-0644(98)70146-5.

[21] Bappal B, George M, Nair R, Khusaiby SA, De Silva V. Factitious hypoglycemia: a tale from the Arab world. Pediatrics 2001;107:180–1.

[22] Gray J, Bentovim A. Illness induction syndrome: paper I – A series of 41 children from 37 families identified at The Great Ormond Street Hospital for Children NHS Trust. Child Abuse Negl 1996;20:655–73.

[23] Günter M. Induction, identification or folie à deux? Psychodynamics and genesis of Munchausen syndromes by proxy and false allegations of sexual abuse in adolescents. Med Law 1998;17:359–79.

[24] Greiner MV, Palusci VJ, Keeshin BR, Kearns SC, Sinal SH. A preliminary screening instrument for early detection of medical child abuse. Hosp Pediatr 2013;3:39–44. doi:10.1542/hpeds.2012-0044.

[25] Mash C, Frazier T, Nowacki A, Worley S, Goldfarb J. Development of a risk-stratification tool for medical child abuse in failure to thrive. Pediatrics 2011;128:e1467–73. doi:10.1542/peds.2011-1080.

[26] Fish E, Bromfield L, Higgins D. A new name for Munchausen syndrome by proxy: defining fabricated or induced illness by carers. Melbourne: Australian Institute of Family Studies; 2005.

[27] Lazoritz S. Munchausen by proxy or Meadow's syndrome? Lancet 1987;330:631. doi:10.1016/S0140-6736(87)93025-X.

[28] Lerman P. Münchausen syndrome by proxy or Polle syndrome. Harefuah 1986;110:248–50.

[29] Meadow R, Lennert T. Munchausen by proxy or Polle syndrome: which term is correct? Pediatrics 1984;74:554–6.

[30] Strassburg HM, Peuckert W. Not "Polle syndrome", please. Lancet 1984;1:166.

[31] Burman D, Stevens D. Munchausen family. Lancet 1977;2:456.

[32] Jolfaei A Ghanbari, Isfahani M Nasr, Bidaki R. Folie à deux and delusional disorder by proxy in a family. J Res Med Sci 2011;16:453–5.

[33] Meadow R. What is, and what is not, "Munchausen syndrome by proxy"? Arch Dis Child 1995;72:534–8.

[34] Bennett AMD, Bennett SMV, Prinsley PR, Wickstead M. Spitting in the ear: a falsified disease using video evidence. J Laryngol Otol 2005;119:926–7. doi:10.1258/002221505774783502.

[35] Bryk M, Siegel PT. My mother caused my illness: the story of a survivor of Munchausen by proxy syndrome. Pediatrics 1997;100:1–7.

[36] Rosenberg DA. Munchausen syndrome by proxy: medical diagnostic criteria. Child Abuse Negl 2003;27:421–30. doi:10.1016/S0145-2134(03)00029-2.

[37] Mayo Clinic Staff. Factitious Disorder: Tests and Diagnosis. Mayo Clin 2014. https://s0.2mdn.net/5368809/1466022075013/300x600/Invega_Trinza_300x600.html (accessed August 6, 2016).

[38] Jones DPH. The untreatable family. Child Abuse Negl 1987;11:409–20. doi:10.1016/0145-2134(87)90014-7.

[39] Dowling D. The child's experience of Munchhausen syndrome by proxy. J Child Psychother 1998;24:307–26. doi:10.1080/00754179808414819.

[40] Schreier HA, Libow JA. Munchausen by proxy syndrome: a modern pediatric challenge. J Pediatr 1994;125:S110–5. doi:10.1016/S0022-3476(05)82934-8.

[41] Schreier H, Ricci LR. Follow-up of a case of Munchausen by proxy syndrome. J Am Acad Child Adolesc Psychiatry 2002;41:1395–6. doi:10.1097/00004583-200212000-00009.

[42] Kucuker H, Demir T, Oral R. Pediatric condition falsification (Munchausen syndrome by proxy) as a continuum of maternal factitious disorder (Munchausen syndrome). Pediatr Diabetes 2010;11:572–8. doi:10.1111/j.1399-5448.2009.00631.x.

[43] Bajanowski T, Vennemann M, Bohnert M, Rauch E, Brinkmann B, Mitchell EA, et al. Unnatural causes of sudden unexpected deaths initially thought to be sudden infant death syndrome. Int J Legal Med 2005;119:213–6. doi:10.1007/s00414-005-0538-8.

[44] Carpenter RG, Waite A, Coombs RC, Daman-Willems C, McKenzie A, Huber J, et al. Repeat sudden unexpected and unexplained infant deaths: natural or unnatural? Lancet 2005;365:29–35. doi:10.1016/S0140-6736(04)17662-9.

[45] Truman TL, Ayoub CC. Considering suffocatory abuse and Munchausen by proxy in the evaluation of children experiencing apparent life-threatening events and sudden infant death syndrome. Child Maltreat 2002;7:138–48. doi:10.1177/1077559502007002006.

[46] Libow JA. Munchausen by proxy victims in adulthood: a first look. Child Abuse Negl 1995;19:1131–42.

[47] Postlethwaite RJ. Caustic ingestion as a manifestation of fabricated and induced Illness (Munchausen syndrome by proxy). Child Abuse Negl 2010;34:471. doi:10.1016/j.chiabu.2009.11.009.

[48] Sanders MJ. Munchausen by proxy: assessment and treatment, AACAP; 2012.

[49] Bauer KA. Covert video surveillance of parents suspected of child abuse: the British experience and alternative approaches. Theor Med Bioeth 2004;25:311–27.

[50] Byard RW, Burnell RH. Covert video surveillance in Munchausen syndrome by proxy. Ethical compromise or essential technique? Med J Aust 1994;160:352–6.

[51] Evans D. The investigation of life-threatening child abuse and Munchausen syndrome by proxy. J Med Ethics 1995;21:9–13.

[52] Flannery MT. First, do no harm: the use of covert video surveillance to detect Munchausen syndrome by proxy—an unethical means of "preventing" child abuse. Univ Mich J Law Reform Univ Mich Law Sch 1998;32:105–94.

[53] Brink FW, Thackeray JD. Factitious illness—Red flags for the pediatric emergency medicine physician. Clin Pediatr Emerg Med 2012;13:213–20. doi:10.1016/j.cpem.2012.06.002.

[54] Jureidini JN, Shafer AT, Donald TG. "Munchausen by proxy syndrome": not only pathological parenting but also problematic doctoring? Med J Aust 2003;178:130–2.

[55] Sugar JA, Belfer M, Israel E, Herzog DB. A 3-year-old boy's chronic diarrhea and unexplained death. J Am Acad Child Adolesc Psychiatry 1991;30:1015–21. doi:10.1097/00004583-199111000-00023.

[56] Zitelli B, Seltman M, Shannon R. Munchausen's syndrome by proxy and its professional participants. Am J Dis Child 1987;141:1095–8. doi:10.1001/archpedi.1987.04460100073029.

[57] Carek DJ. The Munchausen by proxy controversy. J Am Acad Child Adolesc Psychiatry 1995;34:261–261. doi:10.1097/00004583-199503000-00001.

[58] Perman CM. The suspicious physician – legal protections and ramifications for the medical community in identifying and treating Munchausen syndrome by proxy. Health Care Law Mon 2008;2008:2–7.

[59] Kilic SC, Butun C, Beyaztas FY, Ozen B, Sahin RT, Caglar FF. A case of Munchausen syndrome by proxy presenting with epistaxis. Turk Arch Pediatr 2012;47:226–7.

[60] Loo PY, Yap F. Unwitnessed sulphonylurea poisoning in a healthy toddler. Eur J Pediatr 2010;169:1409–12. doi:10.1007/s00431-010-1219-2.

[61] Owen L, Ellis M, Shield J. Deliberate sulphonylurea poisoning mimicking hyperinsulinaemia of infancy. Arch Dis Child 2000;82:392–3.

[62] Tsai H-L, Yang L-Y, Chin T-W, Chen P-H, Yen H-J, Liu C-S, et al. Child abuse in medical setting presenting as gross hematuria: diagnosis by DNA short tandem repeats. Pediatrics 2012;130:e224–9. doi:10.1542/peds.2011-3271.

[63] Ali SN, Ali AN, Ali MN. Munchausen syndrome by proxy: the overlooked diagnosis. J Ayub Med Coll Abbottabad 2015;27:489–91.

[64] Gehlawat P, Gehlawat VK, Singh P, Gupta R. Munchausen syndrome by proxy: an alarming face of child abuse. Indian J Psychol Med 2015;37:90–2. doi:10.4103/0253-7176.150850.

[65] Green RP, Hollander AS, Thevis M, Thomas A, Dietzen DJ. Detection of surreptitious administration of analog insulin to an 8-week-old infant. Pediatrics 2010;125:e1236–40. doi:10.1542/peds.2009-2273.

[66] Narang T, Kanwar AJ, Kumaran MS, Singh SM. Munchausen by proxy in a family. Indian J Dermatol Venereol Leprol 2012;78:748–50. doi:10.4103/0378-6323.102377.

[67] Rabbone I, Galderisi A, Tinti D, Ignaccolo MG, Barbetti F, Cerutti F. Case report: when an induced illness looks like a rare disease. Pediatrics 2015;136:e1361–5. doi:10.1542/peds.2014–4165.

[68] Vadysinghe AN, Dayaratne KMPL. A case of Munchausen syndrome by proxy: is it a misdiagnosis? Sri Lanka J Forensic Med Sci Law 2015;5:3–7.

[69] Foto Özdemir D, Gökler B, Evinç SG, Balseven Odabası A. A case of Munchausen syndrome by proxy in the context of folie a famille. Türk Psikiyatri Derg Turk J Psychiatry 2013;24:275–9.

[70] Barker LH, Howell RJ. Munchausen syndrome by proxy in false allegations of child sexual abuse: legal implications. Bull Am Acad Psychiatry Law 1994;22:499–510.

[71] McClure RJ, Davis PM, Meadow SR, Sibert JR. Epidemiology of Munchausen syndrome by proxy, non-accidental poisoning, and non-accidental suffocation. Arch Dis Child 1996;75:57–61.

[72] Tamay Z, Akcay A, Kilic G, Peykerli G, Devecioglu E, Ones U, et al. Corrosive poisoning mimicking cicatricial pemphigoid: Munchausen by proxy. Child Care Health Dev 2007;33:496–9. doi:10.1111/j.1365-2214.2007.00731.x.

[73] Black D. The extended Munchausen syndrome: a family case. Br J Psychiatry J Ment Sci 1981;138:466–9.

[74] Shapiro M, Nguyen M. Psychological sequelae of Munchausen's syndrome by proxy. Child Abuse Negl 2011;35:87–8. doi:10.1016/j.chiabu.2010.10.005.

[75] Wagner C, Bowers W. Cardiomyopathy in a child induced by intentional ipecac poisoning. Air Med J 2006;25:236–7. doi:10.1016/j.amj.2006.06.006.

[76] Deimel IV GW, Burton MC, Raza SS, Lehman JS, Lapid MI, Bostwick JM. Munchausen syndrome by proxy: an adult dyad. Psychosomatics 2012;53:294–9. doi:10.1016/j.psym.2011.04.006.

[77] Criddle L. Monsters in the closet: Munchausen syndrome by proxy. Crit Care Nurse 2010;30:46–55. doi:10.4037/ccn2010737.

[78] Steinschneider A. Prolonged apnea and the sudden infant death syndrome: clinical and laboratory observations. Pediatrics 1972;50:646–54.

[79] Jenny C, Isaac R. The relation between child death and child maltreatment. Arch Dis Child 2006;91:265–9. doi:10.1136/adc.2004.066696.

[80] Denny SJ, Grant CC, Pinnock R. Epidemiology of Munchausen syndrome by proxy in New Zealand. J Paediatr Child Health 2001;37:240–3.

[81] National Organization for Rare Disorders. NORD Guide to Rare Disorders. Lippincott Williams & Wilkins; Philadelphia, PA 2003.

[82] Al-Owain M, Al-Zaidan H, Al-Hashem A, Kattan H, Al-Dowaish A. Munchausen syndrome by proxy mimicking as Gaucher disease. Eur J Pediatr 2010;169:1029–32. doi:10.1007/s00431-009-1127-5.

[83] Araníbar H, Cerda M. Hypoglycemic seizure in Munchausen-by-proxy syndrome. Pediatr Emerg Care 2005;21:378–9.

[84] Babcock J, Hartman K, Pedersen A, Murphy M, Alving B. Rodenticide-induced coagulopathy in a young child. A case of Munchausen syndrome by proxy. Am J Pediatr Hematol Oncol 1993;15:126–30.

[85] Bader AA, Kerzner B. Ipecac toxicity in "Munchausen syndrome by proxy." Ther Drug Monit 1999;21:259–60.

[86] Barros AJS, Rosa RG, Telles LE de B, Taborda JGV. Atempted serial neonaticides: case report and a brief review of the literature. J Forensic Sci 2016;61:280-283. doi:10.1111/1556–4029.12873.

[87] Bartsch C, Ribe M, Schutz H, Weigand N, Weiler G. Munchausen syndrome by proxy (MSBP): an extreme form of child abuse with a special forensic challenge. Forensic Sci Int 2003;137:147–151.

[88] Baskin DE, Stein F, Coats DK, Paysse EA. Recurrent conjunctivitis as a presentation of Munchausen syndrome by proxy. Ophthalmology 2003;110:1582–4. doi:10.1016/S0161-6420(03)00489-5.

[89] Ben-Chetrit E, Melmed RN. Recurrent hypoglycaemia in multiple myeloma: a case of Munchausen syndrome by proxy in an elderly patient. J Intern Med 1998;244:175–8.

[90] Berkner P, Kastner T, Skolnick L. Chronic ipecac poisoning in infancy: a case report. Pediatrics 1988;82:384–6.

[91] Carlson J, Fernlund P, Ivarsson S-A, Jakobsson I, Neiderud J, Nilsson K, et al. Munchausen syndrome by proxy: an unexpected cause of severe chronic diarrhoea in a child. Acta Pædiatrica 1994;83:119–21. doi:10.1111/j.1651-2227.1994.tb12967.x.

[92] Chodorowsk Z, Anand JS, Porzezińska B, Markiewicz A. Consciousness disturbances: a case report of Munchausen by proxy syndrome in an elderly patient. Przegląd Lek 2003;60:307–8.

[93] Clark RF, Sage TA, Tunget C, Manoguerra AS. Delayed onset lorazepam poisoning successfully reversed by flumazenil in a child. Case report and review of the literature. Pediatr Emerg Care 1995;11:32–4.

[94] Clin B, Ferrant O, Dupont C, Papin F. Recurrent caustic esophagitis: a clinical form of Münchausen syndrome by proxy. Child Abuse Negl 2009;33:293–5. doi:10.1016/j.chiabu.2008.09.007.

[95] Colletti RB, Wasserman RC. Recurrent infantile vomiting due to intentional ipecac poisoning. J Pediatr Gastroenterol Nutr 1989;8:394–6.

[96] Cooper CP, Kamath KR. A toddler with persistent vomiting and diarrhoea. Eur J Pediatr 1998;157:775–6.

[97] D'Avanzo M, Santinelli R, Tolone C, Bettinelli A, Bianchetti MG. Concealed administration of frusemide simulating Bartter syndrome in a 4.5-year-old boy. Pediatr Nephrol Berl Ger 1995;9:749–50.

[98] Day L, Kelly C, Reed G, Andersen JM, Keljo JM. Fatal cardiomyopathy: suspected child abuse by chronic ipecac administration. Vet Hum Toxicol 1989;31:255–7.

[99] Dejoie T, Ramos E, Baron S, Bach-Ngohou K, Masson D. Contribution of the laboratory in hypoglycemia diagnosis induced by insulin administration in a 2-year-old girl. Ann Biol Clin (Paris) 2008;66:82–6. doi:10.1684/abc.2007.0182.

[100] Devore CD, Ulshen MH, Cross RE. Phenolphthalein laxatives and factitious diarrhea. Clin Pediatr (Phila) 1982;21:573–4.

[101] Dine MS, McGovern ME. Intentional poisoning of children—an overlooked category of child abuse: report of seven cases and review of the literature. Pediatrics 1982;70:32–5.

[102] Edidin DV, Farrell EE, Gould VE. Factitious hyperinsulinemic hypoglycemia in infancy: diagnostic pitfalls. Clin Pediatr (Phila) 2000;39:117–9.

[103] Feldman KW, Christopher DM, Opheim KB. Munchausen syndrome/bulimia by proxy: ipecac as a toxin in child abuse. Child Abuse Negl 1989;13:257–61.

[104] Fenton AC, Wailoo MP, Tanner MS. Severe failure to thrive and diarrhoea caused by laxative abuse. Arch Dis Child 1988;63:978.

[105] Friedman EM. Caustic ingestions and foreign body aspirations: an overlooked form of child abuse. Ann Otol Rhinol Laryngol 1987;96:709–12.

[106] Giurgea I, Ulinski T, Touati G, Sempoux C, Mochel F, Brunelle F, et al. Factitious hyperinsulinism leading to pancreatectomy: severe forms of Munchausen syndrome by proxy. Pediatrics 2005;116:e145–8. doi:10.1542/peds.2004-2331.

[107] Glatstein M, Garcia-Bournissen F, Scolnik D, Koren G, Finkelstein Y. Hypoglycemia in a healthy toddler. Ther Drug Monit 2009;31:173–7. doi:10.1097/FTD.0b013e318197b7d7.

[108] Goebel J, Gremse DA, Artman M. Cardiomyopathy from ipecac administration in Munchausen syndrome by proxy. Pediatrics 1993;92:601–3.

[109] Hvizdala EV, Gellady AM. Intentional poisoning of two siblings by prescription drugs. An unusual form of child abuse. Clin Pediatr (Phila) 1978;17:480–2.

[110] Johnson JE, Carpenter BL, Benton J, Cross R, Eaton LA Jr, Rhoads JM. Hemorrhagic colitis and pseudomelanosis coli in ipecac ingestion by proxy. J Pediatr Gastroenterol Nutr 1991;12:501–6.

[111] Jones JG, Butler HL, Hamilton B, Perdue JD, Stern HP, Woody RC. Munchausen syndrome by proxy. Child Abuse Negl 1986;10:33–40.

[112] Kaminer Y, Robbins DR. Insulin misuse: a review of an overlooked psychiatric problem. Psychosomatics 1989;30:19–24. doi:10.1016/S0033-3182(89)72313-6.

[113] Krebs MO, Bouden A, Lôo H, Olié JP. Münchausen syndrome by proxy between two adults. Presse Médicale Paris Fr 1983 1996;25:583–6.

[114] Lansky LL. An unusual case of childhood chloral hydrate poisoning. Am J Dis Child 1974;127:275–6.

[115] Lasala GS, Vearrier D, Boroughf WJ, Osterhoudt KC. Munchausen syndrome by proxy due to tetrahydrozoline poisoning. Clin Toxicol 2014;52:746.

[116] Lorber J. Unexplained episodes of coma in a two-year-old. Lancet Lond Engl 1978;2:472–3.

[117] Lorber J, Reckless JP, Watson JB. Nonaccidental poisoning: the elusive diagnosis. Arch Dis Child 1980;55:643–7.

[118] Lyall EG, Stirling HF, Crofton PM, Kelnar CJ. Albuminuric growth failure. A case of Munchausen syndrome by proxy. Acta Paediatr 1992;81:373–6.

[119] Mahesh VK, Stern HP, Kearns GL, Stroh SE. Application of pharmacokinetics in the diagnosis of chemical abuse in Münchausen syndrome by proxy. Clin Pediatr (Phila) 1988;27:243–6. doi:10.1177/000992288802700507.

[120] Manikoth P, Subramanyan R, Menon S, Al Khusaiby SM. A child with cardiac arrhythmia and convulsions. Lancet 1999;354:2046.

[121] Marks V, Teale JD. Hypoglycemia: factitious and felonious. Endocrinol Metab Clin North Am 1999;28:579–601.

[122] Marks V. Murder by insulin: suspected, purported and proven—a review. Drug Test Anal 2009;1:162–176. doi:10.1002/dta.38.

[123] McClung HJ, Murray R, Braden NJ, Fyda J, Myers RP, Gutches L. Intentional ipecac poisoning in children. Am J Dis Child 1988;142:637–9.

[124] McSweeney JJ, Hoffman RP. Munchausen's syndrome by proxy mistaken for IDDM. Diabetes Care 1991;14:928–9.

[125] Mehl AL, Coble L, Johnson S. Munchausen syndrome by proxy: a family affair. Child Abuse Negl 1990;14:577–85.

[126] Mullins ME, Cristofani CB, Warden CR, Cleary JF. Amitriptyline-associated seizures in a toddler with Munchausen-by-proxy. Pediatr Emerg Care 1999;15:202–5.

[127] Pickering LK, Kohl S. Munchausen syndrome by proxy. Am J Dis Child 1981;135:288–9. doi:10.1001/archpedi.1981.02130270080034.

[128] Proesmans W, Sina JK, Debucquoy P, Renoirte AM, Eeckels R. Recurrent acute renal failure due to nonaccidental poisoning with glafenin in a child. Clin Nephrol 1981;16:207–10.

[129] Rivenes SM, Bakerman PR, Miller MB. Intentional caffeine poisoning in an infant. Pediatrics 1997;99:736–7. doi:10.1542/peds.99.5.736.

[130] Rogers D, Tripp J, Bentovim A, Robinson A, Berry D, Goulding R. Papers and originals. Non-accidental poisoning: an extended syndrome of child abuse. Br Med J 1976;1:793–6.

[131] Rogers R. Diagnostic, explanatory, and detection models of Munchausen by proxy: extrapolations from malingering and deception. Child Abuse Negl 2004;28:225–38.

[132] Santangelo WC, Richey JE, Rivera L, Fordtran JS. Surreptitious ipecac administration simulating intestinal pseudo-obstruction. Ann Intern Med 1989;110:1031–2. doi:10.7326/0003-4819-110-12-1031.

[133] Schneider DJ, Perez A, Knilamus TE, Daniels SR, Bove KE, Bonnell H. Clinical and pathologic aspects of cardiomyopathy from ipecac administration in Munchausen's syndrome by proxy. Pediatrics 1996;97:902–6.

[134] Souid AK, Korins K, Keith D, Dubansky S, Sadowitz PD. Unexplained menorrhagia and hematuria: a case report of Munchausen's syndrome by proxy. Pediatr Hematol Oncol 1993;10:245–8.

[135] Su E, Shoykhet M, Bell MJ. Severe hypernatremia in a hospitalized child: Munchausen by proxy. Pediatr Neurol 2010;43:270–3. doi:10.1016/j.pediatrneurol.2010.05.002.

[136] Sutphen JL, Saulsbury FT. Intentional ipecac poisoning: Munchausen syndrome by proxy. Pediatrics 1988;82:453–6.

[137] Tessa C, Mascalchi M, Matteucci L, Gavazzi C, Domenici R. Permanent brain damage following acute clonidine poisoning in Munchausen by proxy. Neuropediatrics 2001;32:90–2. doi:10.1055/s-2001-13881.

[138] Türkmen Z, Ziyalar N, Tari I, Mercan S, Kayiran SM, Sener D, et al. Toxicological evaluation of two children diagnosed as Munchausen syndrome by proxy. Turk J Pediatr 2012;54:283–6.

[139] Vennemann B, Perdekamp MG, Weinmann W, Faller-Marquardt M, Pollak S, Brandis M. A case of Munchausen syndrome by proxy with subsequent suicide of the mother. Forensic Sci Int 2006;158:195–9. doi:10.1016/j.forsciint.2005.07.014.

[140] Verity CM, Winckworth C, Burman D, Stevens D, White RJ. Polle syndrome: children of Munchausen. Br Med J 1979;2:422–3.

[141] Watson JB, Davies JM, Hunter JL. Nonaccidental poisoning in childhood. Arch Dis Child 1979;54:143–4.

[142] White ST, Voter K, Perry J. Surreptitious warfarin ingestion. Child Abuse Negl 1985;9:349–52. doi:10.1016/0145-2134(85)90031-6.

[143] Yesilkaya E, Akin O, Sari E, Macit E, Akar C, Gun H. A rare reason of hyperinsulinism: Munchausen syndrome by proxy. ESPE Abstr 2015;84:686.

[144] Yonge O, Haase M. Munchausen syndrome and Munchausen syndrome by proxy in a student nurse. Nurse Educ 2004;29:166–9.

[145] Zahavi I, Shaffer EA, Gall DG. Child abuse with laxatives. Can Med Assoc J 1982;127:512–3.

[146] Zylstra RG, Miller KE, Stephens WE. Munchausen syndrome by proxy: a clinical vignette. Prim Care Companion J Clin Psychiatry 2000;2:42–4.

[147] Manoguerra AS, Cobaugh DJ. Guideline on the use of ipecac syrup in the out-of-hospital management of ingested poisons. Clin Toxicol Phila Pa 2005;43:1–10.

[148] Blyth CC, Russell S, Zwi KJ, Taitz J, Fairley M, Post JJ. Munchausen syndrome by proxy and recurrent polymicrobial bacteremia. Pediatr Infect Dis J 2007;26:191. doi:10.1097/01.inf.0000253951.84015.70.

[149] Yalndağ-Öztürk N, Erkek N, Sirinoğlu MB. Think again: first do no harm. Pediatr Emerg Care 2015;31:720–1. doi:10.1097/PEC.0000000000000363.

[150] Schreier H. On the importance of motivation in Munchausen by proxy: the case of Kathy Bush. Child Abuse Negl 2002;26:537–49.

[151] Foto Özdemir D, Yalçın SS, Zeki A, Yurdakök K, Özusta S, Köse A, et al. Munchausen syndrome by proxy presented as recurrent respiratory arrest and thigh abscess: a case study and overview. Turk J Pediatr 2013;55:337–43.

[152] De Sousa A. Trichotillomania by proxy. Int J Trichology 2015;7:24–5. doi:10.4103/0974-7753.153452.

[153] Demircioglu F, Bekdas M, Goksugur SB, Gunes C, Yildirim O. A rare reason in an infant who presented with recurrent bleeding: Munchausen by proxy syndrome. J Med Cases 2014;5:385–7. doi:10.14740/jmc.v5i7.1289.

[154] Jain S, Kumar R, Mehta P, Bhuria J. Munchausen syndrome by proxy masquerading as pyoderma gangrenosum. Indian J Paediatr Dermatol 2014;15:123. doi:10.4103/2319-7250.143667.

[155] Ragaisis K. When the system works: rescuing a child from Munchausen's syndrome by proxy. J Child Adolesc Psychiatr Nurs Off Publ Assoc Child Adolesc Psychiatr Nurses Inc 2004;17:173–6.

[156] Liebson R. Munchausen's role in the strange case of Lacey Spears. Lohud.com 2015.

[157] Artingstall K. Practical Aspects of Munchausen by Proxy and Munchausen Syndrome Investigation. CRC Press; Boca Raton, FL. 1998.

[158] Graeber C. The Good Nurse: A True Story of Medicine, Madness, and Murder. Grand Central Publishing; New York, NY. 2013.

[159] Larimore R, Goldstein D. The Sad, Scary Saga of Justina Pelletier. Slate; 2014. http://www.slate.com/blogs/xx_factor/2014/03/27/justina_pelletier_ruling_boston_children_s_hospital_and_judge_perform_parent.html

[160] Conway Rand D. Book review – "Hurting for love: Munchausen by proxy syndrome." IPT J 1993;5.

[161] Mahoney P. Justina Pelletier Sues Boston Children's Hospital and Alice Newton for Civil Rights Violations and Medical Malpractice 2016. http://christiannewswire.com/news/9980877476.html (accessed August 7, 2016).

[162] Wen P. Alice Newton, Pediatrician is at the Center of Storms on Child Abuse. Boston Globe; Massachusetts, USA. 2015. https://www.bostonglobe.com/metro/2015/11/03/alice-newton-pediatrician-both-admired-and-reviled/f9n28Ni0EvoouJgesk5Z5I/story.html

[163] Jardine C. Has Sally Clark's case changed attitudes to infant death? 2008.

[164] Clark S, Le Fanu J. Roy Meadow. Lancet 2005;366:449–50.

[165] The Royal Statistical Society. Letter from the President to the Lord Chancellor regarding the use of statistical evidence in court cases 2002.

[166] Sir Roy Meadow struck off by GMC. BBC 2005. http://news.bbc.co.uk/2/hi/health/4685511.stm

[167] Chatfield M. Institutionalized Persuasion. CreateSpace Independent Publishing Platform; North Charleston, SC. 2014.

[168] Aswegan AL. Our Ethical Duty Is to Relieve Pain and Suffering. ACEP News; 2007.

[169] Runyan C. Using the Haddon matrix: introducing the third dimension. Inj Prev 1998;4:302–7.

[170] Haddon W. Options for the prevention of motor vehicle crash injury. Isr J Med Sci 1980;16:45–65.

[171] Dowd MD, Keenan HT, Bratton SL. Epidemiology and prevention of childhood injuries. Crit Care Med 2002;30:S385–92.

[172] Mace SE, Gerardi MJ, Dietrich AM, Knazik SR, Mulligan-Smith D, Sweeney RL, et al. Injury prevention and control in children. Ann Emerg Med 2001;38:405–14. doi:10.1067/mem.2001.115882.

Chapter 3

Promoting Patient-Centered Care in Chronic Disease

Ana Monteiro Grilo,
Margarida Custódio dos Santos,
Ana Isabel Gomes and Joana Santos Rita

Additional information is available at the end of the chapter

http://dx.doi.org/10.5772/67380

Abstract

Nowadays, many people around the world are seeing their lives being shattered and even shortened due to one or more chronic conditions. Chronic illness is a dynamic ongoing process that is determined by a complexity of factors. Patient literacy, motivation, emotional well-being, and resources play an important role on patient adaption and are important challenges for healthcare providers. A systematic patient-centered approach that enables chronic patients to play an active role in their condition management and in the decision-making process on a day-to-day basis is required. However, some studies show that health professionals do not always guide their actions by Patient-centered orientation, either by personal issues or by professional and/or institutional barriers. The present chapter aimed to provide a comprehensive approach to patient-centered care in chronic disease and offer a structured guideline as a tool for formal academic education in chronic patient-centered care. This chapter is structured in five sections: (1) Chronic disease: the challenge of the twenty-first century, (2) The patient with a chronic disease, (3) Patient-centered care in chronic diseases, (4) Issues and barriers to achieve patient-centered care, and (5) Guide tool for health professionals' training and education in patient-centered care.

Keywords: patient care, chronic disease, patient empowerment, medical students, health professionals

1. Introduction

Patient-centered care is defined as the professional's attitude during healthcare that is closely congruent with a responsive to patient's wants, needs, and preferences [1]. Although patients differ in their preferences and interaction styles, the patient-centered style has been associated with higher rates of satisfaction, better adherence, and better treatment, particularly in the management of chronic illness [2]. Effective chronic disease management involves continued and coordinated action by the patient and the physician: dynamic partnership with mutual responsibilities and accountabilities.

Nevertheless, some studies conclude that health professionals do not always guide their actions by patient-centered orientation, either by personal issues (e.g., personality characteristics, development of specific communication skills) or by professional and/or institutional barriers [3]. Training health professionals, either during the academic years or in postgraduate courses, can promote the change that is required to accomplish patient centeredness.

The present chapter aimed to provide a comprehensive approach to patient-centered care in chronic disease and offer a structured guideline as a tool for health professionals' training and education in patient-centered care. It will be structured in five sections: (1) Chronic disease: the challenge of the twenty-first century, (2) The patient with a chronic disease, (3) Patient-centered care in chronic diseases, (4) Issues and barriers to achieve patient-centered care, and (5) Guide tool for health professionals' training and education in patient-centered care.

2. Chronic diseases: the challenge of the twenty-first century

The World Health Organization (WHO) defines chronic illnesses as diseases of long duration and generally slow progression. These diseases can usually be controlled but not cured and include persistent and repeated health problems, gradual changes over time, and an asynchronous evolution [4]. Many people around the world are seeing their lives being shattered and even shortened due to one or more chronic conditions [5]. Noncommunicable diseases such as diabetes mellitus, heart disease, obesity, chronic respiratory diseases, and cancer are among the most common [6, 7]. These diseases are the leading cause of death among adults, as well as mortality rates due to them in middle-aged people are higher in some high-income countries [8]. In 2012, about half of adult population had one or more chronic disease, and one of four adults had two or more chronic conditions [9]. Chronic diseases are major causes for disability, including chronic pain, motor and sensory dysfunction, blindness, lower limb amputation, and impaired functioning. In addition, chronic conditions are not only the principal cause for the increased costs in the healthcare system but also for the social costs, like absenteeism at work and decreased productivity [7]. Because of an aging population and the adoption of unhealthy lifestyles, chronic diseases are estimated to grow even further in the next decades. Therefore, it is not surprising that WHO considered chronic conditions the healthcare challenge of this century.

The principal causes of chronic diseases have been identified and well established. Age and hereditary are the only non-modifiable risk factors; in almost all developed countries, most common causes are modifiable, as unhealthy diet and excessive energy intake, tobacco use, physical inactivity, and alcohol abuse [8].

Chronic disease can impact quality of life and daily activities and should require ongoing actions on a long-term basis [10] (**Table 1**). Often, people living with chronic disease face significant life

Dimensions	Examples
Personal	Age, gender
Sensorial	Pain, fatigue, incontinence, joint swelling
Emotional	Anxiety, depression, anger, distress
Cognitive	Negative thoughts, dealing with uncertainty about future, request for information on disease and treatments
Behavioral	Difficulties in activities of daily life, problems with mobility and balance, sleep problems, functional restrictions, medication management
Social	Discrimination, adjustment or end of career, changes in personal relationships
Self/identity	Changes in self-image and self-esteem
Healthcare	More contact with health professionals

Table 1. Experience of chronic disease (adapted from Ref. [10]).

changes and deal with constant threats to their personal health [11]. Most of them must manage daily symptoms, special diets, physical exercise plans, adherence to medication regimens, and systematic monitoring to identify new problems. Each person is affected in a different way by chronic disease; experiences diverge according to personal (e.g., coping strategies), contextual (e.g., access to health systems), and physical (e.g., symptoms) contexts [10].

As indicated in **Table 1**, patients with chronic disease face significant stresses in managing their illness [11] that go far beyond the functional impairments. Therefore, the major goal for healthcare system, and particularly for health professionals, is to address the needs of chronic patients and their care [12].

Nowadays, with effective behavior change efforts and adherence to medication regimens, chronic diseases and their consequences can often be better managed [8, 13]. However, the traditional paternalistic model of care focused on the control of acute symptoms shows itself inadequate to meet the challenge of chronic disease and particularly the needs of chronic patients [14]. A systematic patient-centered approach that enables chronic patients to play an active role in their condition management and in the decision-making process on a day-to-day basis is required [8].

3. The patient with a chronic disease

Patient adaptation to illness has been found to be associated with patient engagement to treatment [15]. Despite differences among patients, studies revealed that the majority of patients and families wish to be more active and involved in treatment decisions and procedures [16]. This involvement, the amount of information, and the development of competencies that usually came along with it may indeed help patients to succeed dealing with disease and treatment's challenges.

Currently, chronic patients (and their families) are, mostly, their own primary healthcare provider. Although they receive support and counselling from health professionals, most patients live the major part of their lives outside of health institutions, they work and have their families. Regarding their illness, patients are expected to motorize their symptoms, to make decisions about adherence behaviors, often to follow complex treatment regimens, to make decisions about when they need to seek professional care, and to make necessary life changes to reach or maintain better health outcomes. Effective self-management is, then, considered critical to meet the needs of people living with long-term conditions. Self-management has been defined as "the care taken by individuals towards their own health and well-being: it comprises the actions they take to lead a healthy lifestyle; to meet their social, emotional and psychological needs; to care for their long-term condition; and to prevent further illness or accidents" [17].

Some factors related to the patient have been repeatedly highlighted to influence the way patient's cope with this challenges.

3.1. Patient literacy

Health literacy respects to the ability to read, understand, and act upon health information and has been associated with the skills for making appropriate health decisions [18]. Receiving clear information and education increases patient understanding of the disease implications. On the other hand, information about treatment procedures enhances patient's auto-efficacy and self-confidence.

Three distinct levels or purposes of health literacy have been identified: *functional*, basic skills in reading and writing necessary for effective functioning in a health context; *interactive*, more advanced cognitive literacy and social skills that enable active participation in healthcare; and *critical*, the ability to critically analyze and use information to participate in actions that overcome structural barriers to health [16].

A systematic review by Berkman and colleagues to determine whether low health literacy is related to the poorer use of healthcare, outcomes, costs, and disparities in health outcomes among persons of all ages found that low literacy was associated with poorer health outcomes and the poorer use of healthcare services [19]. Association between good level of health literacy and treatment outcomes, patient satisfaction, and better quality of care was also found in recent studies [20, 21].

3.2. Patient willingness and motivation

Studies show that, in general, patients wish some degree of participation on their care [22, 23]. Nevertheless, despite the evident benefits, not all patients feel motivated to participate in their care, to adhere to medical recommendations, or to change lifestyles or health behaviors that are key stones for their treatment. Hibbard and colleagues, in a study with adults aged 45–97 years old with chronic diseases, found that only 22% adopted more involved and active behaviors to participate in their treatment, 12% do not think that they must play an active role in their own health believing that they are just recipients of healthcare, 29% do not have enough information or understanding about their clinical situation and their treatment, and 37% have the understanding but not the confidence to be more involved [24].

In a qualitative study that aimed to explore patients' and practitioners' views on factors influencing engagement in self-management in the context of multimorbidity, with a sample drawn from four general practices in Greater Manchester, motivation emerged as one of the three themes that captured patients' and professionals' views. In this study, motivation drew on understandings that successful self-management was partly contingent on patients' belief and expectation that self-management would improve their health and how low mood can negatively influence patients' capacity and sense of responsibility for self-management [25].

Regarding adherence, in a study focused in the relation between physiotherapist's attitudes and patient adherence, Chan and colleagues found that patient's treatment motivation mediated the relationship between physiotherapist's autonomy supportive behaviors and rehabilitation adherence [26]. Increasing patient motivation through motivational strategies and motivational interviewing can be used to reduce resistance and improve the odds of achieving positive clinical outcomes among noncompliant/resistant patients [27]. Highlighting the importance of motivation on patient adherence [28], a meta-analysis of systematic reviews about the effectiveness of adherence interventions published between 1990 and 2005 found that interventions focused on behavioral interventions that used incentives and patient motivation were among the most effective to promote adherence.

3.3. Patient emotional disorders

Depression is frequently associated with chronic conditions and, if untreated, can adversely affect the course of the disease and limit effective treatment for the chronic condition [29]. For instance, depression was found in 27% of diabetic population compared with 17% in the non-diabetic population. Those patients with diabetes and depression experienced an impact with a large effect size on quality of life, as compared with those who suffered diabetes and who were not depressed [30]. In another study, depression coexisting with diabetes was associated with poorer glycemic control, increased risk of complications, increased healthcare utilization and costs, increased functional disability, and lost work productivity [31]. There is also some evidence that depression affects self-management. Patients with depressive symptoms (including subclinical depression) were found much less likely to gain in activation and in their self-management behaviors [32].

3.4. Patient resources

Social support refers to the degree to which interpersonal relationships correspond to certain functions of material support, affective, emotional, informative, and positive social interaction [33] and is a multifaceted experience that involves voluntary associations and formal and informal relationships with others [34]. Social support can buffer the negative impact of life events on health and positively influence psychosocial adjustment and self-management of chronic illness [35]. A large amount of studies found associations between social support and clinical and self-management/self-care behaviors [36], health-related quality of life [37, 38], and patient adherence to treatment [39]. Patient's network for social support includes family and friends, social environment, and all health providers [40].

In conclusion, adaptation to chronic illness is a dynamic ongoing process that is determined by a complexity of factors. Evidence has shown that patients are decision-makers that may actively contribute to their own care. Patient literacy, motivation, emotional well-being, and resources play an important role on patient adaption and are important challenges for healthcare providers. These challenges are better attended within the framework of the patient-centered model of care.

4. Patient-centered care in chronic diseases

Chronic disease management demands the adaptation of the patient-centered care model to the changing patients' needs. Hudon and colleagues developed a thematic analysis based on Stewart's[1] model of patient-centered care, based on articles published between 1980 and 2009. They found six major themes: (a) *Starting from the patient's situation,* (b) *Legitimizing the illness experience,* (c) *Acknowledging the patient's expertise,* (d) *Developing an ongoing partnership,* (e) *Offering realistic hope,* and (f) *Providing patients' advocacy in the healthcare system* [2].

4.1. Starting from the patient situation

Chronic patient-centered care requires an extended comprehension of the patient's situation. This theme included two subthemes corresponding to Stewart et al. dimensions *exploring both the disease and the illness* and *understanding the whole person. Exploring both the disease and the illness* means to discover the patient's personal and subjective experience of sickness: worries, feelings, expectations, previous experience of care, health behaviors, and confidence with chronic conditions management, with the same interested as the biological dimensions like physical evaluation and laboratory results.

Understanding the whole person, as the act of being aware of the surrounding circumstances of patient's life, implies the acknowledgment that chronic health meanings could vary with adjacent environments. Stewart and colleagues (2003) recognize that take into account various aspects of the patient's personal and life context allowed health professional's comprehension to the several factors that influence patient's complex dynamic responses to chronic condition [41]. Contextual factors could be proximal and distal to the patient [41]. Proximal factors refer to immediate and specific categories and comprise family, financial security, education, employment, leisure, and social support. Distal factors are related with general and meta-context categories and include community, culture, healthcare system, sociohistorical period, geography, and the media.

4.2. Legitimizing the illness experience

Chronic patient-centered care includes attending to patient's needs, worries, and emotions as grief over their previous skills and allows them to express their concerns related to their

[1]Stewart et al. (2006) model included six components: exploring both the disease and the illness experience, understanding the whole person, finding common ground,incorporating prevention and health promotion, enhancing the patient-doctor relationship, and being realistic.

chronic conditions. By recognizing subjective perceptions and sensations of illness, health professionals formally acknowledge the reality of the patient's experiences and allow the patient to feel that his definition of reality is confirmed [42]. Legitimation helped patient in his/her illness adaptation process and improve patient-health professional relationship. Lehman and colleagues show that patients with chronic fatigue syndrome report more psychological distress and dissatisfaction when physician failed to legitimize their illness [43]. This theme is one of the most important, when improving centered care is a priority.

4.3. Acknowledging patient expertise on his/her own life

One of the central premises of Carl Rogers' patient-centered model is the idea that each patient is the world best expert on himself [44]. Patient's expertise should be acknowledged and respected by the caregiver. In chronic disease, great management of the conditions depends on patient's actions; therefore, all the interactions with health professionals should centered on patients' strengths and challenges on running their disease condition. The development of self-management plans should integrate not only the health professional expertise but also the patient's concerns, priorities, and resources. Usually, patients appreciate being treated as a full member of the health team, as this promotes their sense of control and empowerment [10]. This requires a new empowerment paradigm, with redefinition of patient and health professional roles [45].

4.4. Developing an ongoing partnership

Effective chronic disease management entails an ongoing partnership between patient and health professionals. Partnership refers to both a relationship and a process [10, 35] and promotes patient empowering to take control over his/her situation. Therefore, patients can be involved in their care as an active partner, helping to clarify symptoms and diagnosis, sharing decisions and treatments responsibilities, discussing treatment outcomes and alternatives, and agreeing on a treatment plan. This theme corresponds to two subthemes on Stewart and colleagues model: enhancement of the physician-patient relationship and finding common ground [41].

Mutual respect, trust, and collaborative action are essential ingredients to build and *enhance the patient-physician relationship*. Both patient and health professional need to feel committed to sharing power and responsibility [10]. In chronic disease, physical conditions and patients' preferences and capacities change over time and determine the nature of partnership in which moment. On the other hand, continuity of care is an opportunity to improve the patient-health professional relationship, to empower the patient and to support during the most difficult phases of chronic condition. According to this author, an effective partnership depends on four factors: patient (e.g., stage of adjustment to chronic illness, self-esteem), adjunctive factors (e.g., family support, health service resources), communication process (patient and health professional verbal and no verbal skills), and health professional (e.g., attitudes related to own role, self-awareness).

Finding a common ground is the process by which health professional and patient range a mutual understanding and agreement related to chronic disease (the problem), goals and priorities in management and/or treatment of chronic disease, and roles to be assumed both by patient and health professional [41]. Patient needs, preferences, and beliefs should be respected always.

4.5. Offering realistic hope

This theme emphasizes on hope and support in the context of uncertainty or the inevitable deterioration of chronic conditions and contrasts from Stewart and colleagues (2006) *being realistic* issue. Hope has been identified as a key attribute required for patient adaption to illness and disability [46]. Giving hope tempered with realism allows patients to deal with uncertainty and promotes patient well-being and adaptation. Hope does not suppress negative aspects of the illness but includes and focuses on the positive, less negative, and possible developments that may be considered better outcomes or better patient quality of life [47].

4.6. Providing patients' advocacy in the healthcare system

This theme is new considering Stewart`s model and relates to the health professional's role in guiding the patient through the healthcare system. That means defending their rights, interests and safety. Often, chronic conditions are complex and patients need different levels of care (e.g., physiotherapy), support groups, and community services.

4.7. Over time

The six themes previously described comprise a longitudinal dimension. Patient's situation could change depending on the disease course, life context, and illness experience. On the other hand, patients' expectations, knowledge, and expertise in self-management of his/her chronic conditions could improve (or not) over time and influence patient-health professional relationship. As the disease progresses, values, goals, and preferences must be reassessed and discussed. Even health professional advocacy role should be adjusted to patient desires at a particular time.

5. Issues and barriers to achieve patient-centered care

The WHO (2005) recognizes the potential benefits of chronic patient-centered care but also identifies many challenges when applying this approach [16]. In fact, even when health professionals recognize patient-centered approach as an essential feature in clinical practice, they report difficulties in maintaining these behaviors during care. Personal and professional barriers need to be considered to carry on this challenge.

5.1. Organizational barriers

Time constrains, staff shortage, and work overload are frequently mentioned as major difficulties for a patient-centered care by health professionals [48]. In a study developed by West and colleagues, nurses acknowledge that lack of time frequently compromises their ability to provide clear and complete information to patients and their families, to give effective emotional support, and to offer the appropriate treatment according to patient's clinical needs and safety [49]. The limited time available for medical appointment is also referred by doctors [50, 51] and patients [52] as a barrier to provide information about diagnosis and to discuss treatment options. The impossibility to control physical environment features like temperature or noise can reduce the possibility of health professionals to comply with patient's specific needs during recovery [49]. In addition, a private space that guarantees patient's confidentiality and dignity during medical procedures is a condition difficult to offer in healthcare institutions [49].

5.2. Interpersonal barriers

The lack of a common acknowledgment about the relevance of patient-centered practices in healthcare among professionals' team is mentioned as an important barrier [53]. The health team relationships and the conditions given to the staff to effectively consider patients' perspectives appear to facilitate a more generalized patient-centered attitude. When clinical and personal information about the patient is shared by the health team, the health professionals have major opportunities to make stronger and more consistent decisions about the best interventions toward the patient [54]. A prior and clear definition of the clinical practice role of each health professional regarding patients' care and communication seems to be very useful to overcome difficulties in applying correctly a patient-centered attitude [55].

5.3. Individual barriers

Several studies have highlighted specific health professionals' beliefs and feelings as possible barriers to a more patient-centered attitude. The fear of leading with patient's emotional distress has been identified as an important obstacle for the adoption of relational models that approach nurses from their patients [49, 56]. Nurses feel frequently that the emotional detachment from their work and their patients is essential to keep going emotionally and mentally healthy and to prevent stress and burnout [57].

The professionals' perception of patient roles and responsibilities can also affect their intervention during the medical procedures. In a study presented by Jallinoja and colleagues, nurses and physicians identify patients' willingness to make changes in their lifestyles in a chronic disease context as a barrier to treatment [58]. Pessimistic judgments or unrealistic expectations about patients' abilities to make effective lifestyle changes can compromise medical actions based in promoting empowerment. In a systematic review about barriers to the adoption of a shared decision-making process by physicians, doctors perceived inability to balance patients' preferences with the clinical guidelines available, and they are afraid that the implementation of a shared decision-making process leads to patients' discomfort or threats health professionals' autonomy. Moreover, the perception that shared decision-making practices does not contribute significantly to better patient's outcomes is identified as a possible difficulty [48]. Lack of motivation and difficulties in following a holistic approach are another two important problems referred by nurses

The gap between the "ideal" academically taught and the "real" clinical practice can lead to the withdrawal of patient-centered attitudes and to the adoption of more traditional paternalistic models [59, 60]. During the academic internship and among recently graduated health professionals is evident some inconstancy in orientation assumed toward patients.

That is students and professionals range from focusing exclusively in accomplish procedures and tasks correctly, or accent primary in patients' needs and worries [51, 61, 62]. The newness of the experience endorses lack of confidence and uncertainly, when students have to decide about the right action to implement in specific situations during healthcare [63], and gives more strength to students' preconceptions and stereotypes about patients [62]. In this period, senior colleagues who have responsibilities in tutoring students in their first interactions with patients play an important role as models [64]. However, not always those first clinical experiences are properly supervised [65] nor patient-centered care orientation is defended and practiced by tutors [51, 60, 66]. In this context, students face problems in really translating patient-centered approach into nursing care, because poor or ineffective teaching strategies were used to training patient-centered care skills [67, 68].

5.4. Providing healthcare to specific chronic patient groups

Difficulties in effective communication and patient-centered attitudes seem to exacerbate when healthcare is provided to certain patient groups, namely, patients with intellectual disabilities [69], critically ill patients [70], patients with severe communication impairment [71], elderly [63, 72] and pediatrics patients [73], and cancer patients [55].

6. Guide tool for health professionals' training and education in patient-centered care

Patient-centered care requires competences in communication skills. Nowadays, many medical schools recognize the impact of communication skills and use guidelines to teach and assess these competences during undergraduate medical training [74, 75]. The recent European consensus on learning objectives for a core communication curriculum in healthcare professions [47] states as key tasks: (a) build relationship and develop trust and rapport; (b) elicit information from the patient/problems and concerns; (c) consider the patient's perspective of the illness; (d) give relevant information and explanations; (e) develop shared plan of care; and (f) close the interview and set up next meeting.

Considering the effectiveness of several earlier guidelines about communication skills training in healthcare professional's education, namely, the Calgary Cambridge [76], the Four Habits Model [77], Kalamazoo Consensus Framework [75], REDE Model Skills Checklist [74], and the Health Professionals Core Communication Curriculum [47], we propose a tool aimed to systematize major dimensions of patient-centered care in chronic illness as defined by Hudon and colleagues into their specific core conditions and respective communication skills, with examples of interactions with the patient (**Table 2**).

Regarding methods for effective training and education of health professionals' students, active learning and reflective learning seem to be the most effective teaching strategies [75]. At the start, core conditions and communication skills have to be explained [76], and evidence of their utility in chronic patient-centered care should be provided. In formal

http://dx.doi.org/10.5772/67380

1. Starting from the patient situation	
Core conditions	Gather information: (a) encourage patients to tell story of problems in own words; (b) explore both the disease and the illness means (scan how each problem affects the patient's life); examine patient beliefs, concerns, and expectations. Enhance patient to talk and express feelings.
Skills	Use **open-ended questions** to initiate patient narrative. Identify patient's problems or subjects that patients desire to discuss with appropriate **open questions**. Use **VIEW** questions [74]: Vital activities: *How does chemotherapy treatment impact on daily routines?* Ideas: *What do you think of talking to our psychologist about the emotional impact of chemotherapy treatment?* Expectations: *You are going to finish your chemotherapy treatment today. What are your expectations about it?* Worries: *What worries you most about chemotherapy treatment side effects?*. **Listen** attentively without interruption, facilitating patient's responses verbally (e.g., *yes; ah, ah; go on; mm-hmm; I see*) and nonverbal (e.g., eye contact, facial expression) facilitation. Attend to **nonverbal cues,** checking out body language and facial expression (e.g., *This seems to be a difficult problem of you…*). **Clarify** statements that are unclear or need amplification, with more specify or yes/no questions (e.g., *Could you explain what you mean by having two bad days?*). **Summarize** patient narrative to verify understanding of what the patient has said (e.g., *So, you feel very tired and you think that your tiredness is not related with the intense work period you have been involved*), and give patient opportunity to correct or add information.
2. Legitimizing the illness experience	
Core conditions	Recognize emotional cues and clarify the emotion (if necessary). Validate patient's views and feelings, avoiding judgments.
Skills	Demonstrate **empathy**, showing interest and care in the patient experience. Communicate understanding and appreciation of patient's feeling or situation, using **SAVE** [74]. Support: *We are going to work together to find better solution to control your pain.* Acknowledge: *The experience you describe during your back pain crisis sound overwhelming.* Validate: *It's very common for people with persistent pain feel exasperated and discouraged like you do.* Emotion naming: *You seem more discouraged today than our last appointment.* Use **no verbal cues** (tone, eye contact, and posture) that show care and concern.
3. Acknowledging patient expertise on their own lives	
Core conditions	Recognize patient's attributes and expertise. Reinforce patient's skills and strengths. Determine how much the patient desire to be included in choices and decisions and clarify your own role as a supporter and a trustful information provider. Negotiate a mutually acceptable plan.
Skills	Use **open-ended questions** to encourage patients to talk about illness, their experience, and their sources of information (e.g., *What do you think are the most difficult task of your treatment? Where did you look for information on your illness?*). **Listen attentively,** allowing patients to complete what they have to say without interruptions. Use **reflection**, to acknowledge what has worked with the patient (e.g., *I see you already exercised three times a day. It is very important for your diabetes to exercise*) and/or his/her resources and strengths (*I realize you are very motivated to change your diet and start eating more health food).* Support patients, using **clarification** questions that help them to rephrase information that is unclear or needs amplification *(e.g., You are saying that having to take that pill worries you. Can you explain a little more?).* Express the importance of patient expertise by **incorporating** patient's opinions, values, and needs in treatment plans (*e.g., Based on your concerns, I think that we should change our initial plan. What is your opinion?*).

		Use **negotiation,** showing respect about patient's needs, expectations, and objectives (*What do you expect form this treatment?),* asking questions and promoting answers that may clarify the object of negotiation (*Can you explain what you meant by having difficulties in think about this diet*?), providing information that allows the discussion of different alternatives, understanding patient limitations (e.g., the resources that are need to implement a specific treatment), highlighting shared points of view and showing pleasure in agreement (*I am very glad that we agree on several issues about your diet plan),* and arranging plans that recurrently reassess decisions and help to adjust them if needed.
4. Developing an ongoing partnership		
Core conditions	Enhancing the patient-physician relationship	Reveal interest in the patient as a person. Develop trust and rapport, accepting legitimacy of patient's views and feeling. Provide support adjusted to the stage of chronic illness.
	Finding common ground	Focus on working collaboratively to meet patient goals. Provide reliable, clear, evidence-based, and individualized information that promotes sharing decision and responsibilities. Use adequate strategies to clarify patient's doubts and to support patient's decisions. Promote the sense of "joining together" with patients in supportive partnerships collaboration to meet patient's goals. Promote patient's sharing information and educate patients on how to reach information and how to motorize treatment outcomes. Develop and use systems to record, communicate, and monitor the implementation of patient's preferences.
Skills	Enhancing the patient-physician relationship	Attend to **patient's privacy, confidentiality, and autonomy**. **Acknowledge difficult situations and challenges** during the chronic illness stages, providing continued, willing, helpful, gentle, supportive care. **Deal kindly** with embarrassing and disturbing issues. Avoid **interrupting** and **respect the silences**. Avoid **direct advice** (*You should…*), **impositions** (*You have to…*), or over, not realistic **tranquilization** (*I'm sure you are going to be fine.*). Consider patient's degree of understanding and language, **avoiding jargons**. Use **BUSTER** [78]. Be prepared: define a plan to manage for specific patient's emotions and practice self-regulation. Use nonjudgmental listening. Six second rule: avoid escalation of conversation. "Tell me more" statements: *Can you tell me more about that worry that you just mentioned now?* Empathize and validate*: It isn't easy to talk about your illness, is it?* Respond with a wish statement: *I wish this treatment had been more effective*
	Finding common ground	**Provide information**, tailoring information to what the patient wants and/or is able to know, using words that show that you prioritize patient information needs, thru categories (e.g. *Let's talk about medication side effects*) and "7C": clear, concise, concrete, correct, coherent, complete, and courteous [79]. Check if the patients would like more information; if necessary, provide **writing or audio-taping information**. Be sure that your information promotes patient's understanding and skills for decision taking. Make **suggestions**, rather than given directives (e.g., *I would like to make a suggestion about your diet*) and **encourage patient to make choices** (e.*g., Let's talk about your alternatives. I think you have three options here…*).

http://dx.doi.org/10.5772/67380

	Check understanding by asking patients **feedback** or **teach back**, asking to, in their own words, tell what you have just explained. Be careful and try not tosound like you are testing your patient (e.g., *We have been talking about your diet. What do you think is the most important information so far, as for instance? Could you explain it back to me? I really want to know if I was clear enough).*
	Encourage questions, stating, e.g., *Your questions are very important for me and four your process,* and use **open-end questions**, eliciting patient's preference and views in relation to treatment options (e.g., *For you what are the main benefits of this treatment? What about surgery?*).
	Reinforce patients for achieving small successes encouraging them to raise expectations about self-efficacy and enhancing involvement in partnership (e.g., *We did so well. Your effort was compensated. I know we can do even more.).*
	Provide **education on patient treatment** by **modeling** and/or delivering **written information and instructions** that promote patient feeling of self-efficacy and encourage patients to build their own capacity for self-management.
5. Offering realistic hope	
Core conditions	Being responsive to patients' concerns emotions and suffering. Being honest and trustful, providing clear update and realistic information. Having a positive attitude toward the diagnosis, the treatment, and the care. Including patient education and capacitation to decrease uncertainty.
Skills	Promote patients' control toward the treatment and their own quality of life by **providing clear and realistic information** that allows patients to reduce uncertainty and to be aware of different alternatives and new developments. Promote patients' positive thinking by using **positive talk.**

Table 2. Guidelines for effective communication with chronic health patients based on patient-centered care principles as defined by Hudon and colleagues [2].

academic education, active patient participation can be achieved either by using actor-simulated patients (sometimes called standardized patients) or by engaging real patient to share their own experiences [80, 81]. Videos can also be used. One good example is the Database of Individual Patient Experience of Illness (DIPEx) [82]. These educational sessions should be an ongoing task in clinical education and must be carefully plan to give space to trainees' reflection. Participants should be able to discuss the skills used and the impact of the trained skills on the patient on health professional and should have the opportunity to obtain feedback on their performance [83].

Moreover, learning and training communication skills should be an ongoing process during academic and professional education and meet the progressively more difficult demands that are placed on students and professionals. Thus, for example, basic communication skills such as welcoming the patient or developing empathy should be the focus of training in the early years. On the other hand, issues such as giving bad news or dealing with emotionally disturbing situations should be integrated into the more advanced years of training.

At the end of the training, participants should be able to use a checklist that helps them to verify if all dimensions of chronic patient-centered care model have been considered during their interaction with patient (**Table 3**).

	Yes/no	Observation
I understand the patient's perspective of his/her situation		
I validated (with empathy) patient's experience and feelings		
I asked and understand what are the patient's main concerns		
I provided information I want to give and that answered patient's needs		
I check that I have responded adequately to the patient's demands		
I encourage patient's skills and strengths		
We shared decision in the level patient's feel comfortable		
I offer realistic hope considering patient situation		

Table 3. Checklist for health professionals' self-evaluation regarding communication and interaction with patients, based on patient-centered care principles as defined by Hudon and colleagues [2].

7. Conclusions

In this chapter, we have described some of the challenges motivated by chronic disease management demands and outlined some core principles of patient-centered care in chronic disease. Promoting a chronic patient-centered approach is likely depending on giving primacy to the subjective aspects of illness, therefore is not a simple matter and must be included in all levels of medical education. Two important next steps concerning the development of chronic patient-centered model must be considered. First, training skills programs must be integrated in preclinical courses and not only in courses of communication as usually. Second, principles of chronic patient-centered model should be applied to a wide variety of chronic diseases, making them tangibly significant to concrete clinical conditions.

Author details

Ana Monteiro Grilo[1*], Margarida Custódio dos Santos[1,2], Ana Isabel Gomes[3] and Joana Santos Rita[4]

*Address all correspondence to: ana.grilo@estesl.ipl.pt

1 Higher School of Health Technology, Polytechnic Institute of Lisbon, Lisbon, Portugal

2 Faculty of Psychology, University of Lisbon, Lisbon, Portugal

3 Lusíadas Lisbon Hospital, Lisbon, Portugal

4 Lisbon Regional Health Administration, Odivelas Health Care Centers, Lisbon, Portugal

http://dx.doi.org/10.5772/67380

References

[1] Laine C, Davidoff F. Patient-centered medicine: a professional evolution. JAMA. 1996;275(2):152-6.

[2] Hudon C, Fortin M, Haggerty J, Loignon C, Lambert M, Poitras ME. Patient-centered care in chronic disease management: a thematic analysis of the literature in family medicine. Patient Education and Counseling. 2012;88(2):170-6.

[3] McCabe C. Nurse–patient communication: an exploration of patients' experiences. Journal of Clinical Nursing. 2004;13(1):41-9.

[4] Bentzen, N, ed. Wonca Dictionary of General/Family Practice. Wonca International Classification Committee: Copenhagen, 2003.

[5] Wu S, Green A. Projection of chronic illness prevalence and cost inflation. Santa Monica, CA: RAND Health; 2000.

[6] Martin C. Chronic disease and illness care. Canadian Family Physician. 2007;53:2086-91.

[7] Mendis S, Armstrong T, Bettcher D, Branca F, Lauer J, Mace C, et al. GLOBAL STATUS REPORT on noncommunicable diseases 2014. Geneva: World Health Organization; 2015.

[8] WHO. Preventing chronic diseases: a vital investment. WHO Global Report. Geneva: WHO; 2005.

[9] Ward B, Schiller J, Goodman R. Multiple chronic conditions among US adults: a 2012 update. Preventing Chronic Disease. 2014;11:130389.

[10] Reynolds F. Communication and clinical effectiveness in rehabilitation. Edinburgh: Elsevier Butterworth Heinemann; 2005.

[11] Boyd CM, Wolff JL, Giovannetti E, Reider L, Weiss C, Xue QL, et al. Health care task difficulty among older adults with multimorbidity. Medical Care. 2014;52(3):S118-25.

[12] Trehearne B, Fishman P, Lin E. Role of the nurse in chronic illness management: making the medical home more effective. Nursing Economics. 2014;32(4):178-84.

[13] McMullen CS, Safford M, Bosworth H, Phansalkar S, Leong A, Fagan M, et al. Patient-centered priorities for improving medication management and adherence. Patient Education and Counseling. 2015;98:102-10.

[14] Brock C, Dost A. Self-care—a real choice: self-care support—a practical option. London: Department of Health; 2005.

[15] Hibbard JH, Greene J. What the evidence shows about patient activation: better health outcomes and care experiences; fewer data on costs. Health Affairs. 2013;32(2):207-14.

[16] Coulter A, Parsons S, Askham J. Policy brief: Where are the patients in decision-making about their own care. WHO 2008 and WHO on behalf of the European Observatory on Health Systems and Policies 2008. Denmark: World Health Organisation; 2008.

[17] Clark N, Becker M, Janz N, Lorig K, Rawkowski W, Anderson L. Self-management of chronic disease by older adults: a review and questions for research. Journal of Aging and Health. 1991;3:3-27.

[18] Nielsen-Bohlman L, Panzer A, Kindig D. Health literacy: a prescription to end confusion. Institute of Medicine of National Academics. Washington, D.C.: National Academies Press; 2004.

[19] Berkman ND, Sheridan SL, Donahue KE, Halpern DJ, Crotty K. Low health literacy and health outcomes: an updated systematic review. Annals of Internal Medicine. 2011;155(2):97-107.

[20] Altin SV, Stock S. The impact of health literacy, patient-centered communication and shared decision-making on patients' satisfaction with care received in German primary care practices. BMC Health Services Research. 2016;16(1):450-60.

[21] Fisher CA, Myers M. Patient education: a win-win opportunity. Nursing Management. 2016;47(3):18-20.

[22] Foot C, Gilburt H, Dunn P, Jabbal J, Seale B, Goodrich J, et al. People in control of their own health and care: the state of involvement. London: The Kings Fund; 2014.

[23] Vahdat S, Hamzehgardeshi L, Hessam S, Hamzehgardeshi Z. Patient involvement in health care decision making: a review. Iranian Red Crescent Medical Journal. 2014; 16(1):e12454.

[24] Hibbard JH, Mahoney ER, Stockard J, Tusler M. Development and testing of a short form of the patient activation measure. Health services research. 2005;40(6p1):1918-30.

[25] Coventry PA, Fisher L, Kenning C, Bee P, Bower P. Capacity, responsibility, and motivation: a critical qualitative evaluation of patient and practitioner views about barriers to self-management in people with multimorbidity. BMC Health Services Research. 2014;14(1):536-48.

[26] Chan DK, Lonsdale C, Ho PY, Yung PS, Chan KM. Patient motivation and adherence to postsurgery rehabilitation exercise recommendations: the influence of physiotherapists' autonomy-supportive behaviors. Archives of Physical Medicine and Rehabilitation. 2009;90(12):1977-82.

[27] Butterworth SW. Influencing patient adherence to treatment guidelines. Journal of Managed Care & Specialty Pharmacy. 2008;14(6 Supp B):21-5.

[28] van Dulmen S, Sluijs E, van Dijk L, de Ridder D, Heerdink R, Bensing J. Patient adherence to medical treatment: a review of reviews. BMC Health Services Research. 2007;7(1):1-13.

[29] Chapman DP, Perry GS, Strine TW. The vital link between chronic disease and depressive disorders. Preventing Chronic Diseases. 2005;2(1):1-10.

[30] Goldney RD, Phillips PJ, Fisher LJ, Wilson DH. Diabetes, depression, and quality of life a population study. Diabetes Care. 2004;27(5):1066-70.

[31] Egede LE. Effect of comorbid chronic diseases on prevalence and odds of depression in adults with diabetes. Psychosomatic Medicine. 2005;67(1):46-51.

[32] Hibbard JH, Mahoney ER, Stock R, Tusler M. Do increases in patient activation result in improved self-management behaviors? Health Services Research. 2007;42(4):1443-63.

[33] Griep RH, Chor D, Faerstein E, Werneck GL, Lopes CS. Social support: scale test-retest reliability in the Pro-Health Study. Cadernos de Saúde Pública. 2003;19(2):625-34.

[34] Bardach SH, Tarasenko YN, Schoenberg NE. The role of social support in multiple morbidity: self-management among rural residents. Journal of Health Care for the Poor and Underserved. 2011;22(3):759-71.

[35] Gallant MP. The influence of social support on chronic illness self-management: a review and directions for research. Health Education & Behavior. 2003;30(2):170-95.

[36] Strom JL, Egede LE. The impact of social support on outcomes in adult patients with type 2 diabetes: a systematic review. Current Diabetes Reports. 2012;12(6):769-81.

[37] Colloca G, Colloca P. The effects of social support on health-related quality of life of patients with metastatic prostate cancer. Journal of Cancer Education. 2016;31(2):244-52.

[38] Degroote S, Vogelaers D, Vandijck DM. What determines health-related quality of life among people living with HIV: an updated review of the literature. Archives of Public Health. 2014;72(1):40-50.

[39] Miller TA, DiMatteo MR. Importance of family/social support and impact on adherence to diabetic therapy. Diabetes Metabolic Syndrome and Obesity: Targets and Therapy. 2013;6(6):421-6.

[40] Neri L, Brancaccio D, Rocca RL, Rossa F, Martini A, Andreucci VE. Social support from health care providers is associated with reduced illness intrusiveness in hemodialysis patients. Clinical Nephrology. 2011;75(2):125-34.

[41] Stewart M, Belle Brown J, Weston W, McWhinney I, McWilliam C, Freeman T. Patientcentered medicine: transforming the clinical method. 2nd ed. Oxford UK: Radcliffe Medical Press Ltd; 2003.

[42] Ware NC. Suffering and the social construction of illness: the delegitimation of illness experience in chronic fatigue syndrome. Medical Anthropology Quarterly. 1992; 6(4):347-61.

[43] Lehman AM, Lehman DR, Hemphill KJ, Mandel DR, Cooper LM. Illness experience, depression, and anxiety in chronic fatigue syndrome. Journal of Psychosomatic Research. 2002;52(6):461-5.

[44] Rogers CR. A theory of therapy, personality, and interpersonal relationships, as developed in the client-centered framework. In: Koch S, editor. Psychology: A Study of a Science.. Vol. 3. New York: McGraw-Hill; 1956. pp. 184-256.

[45] Anderson R, Funnell M. Patient empowerment: reflections on the challenge of fostering the adoption of a new paradigm. Patient Education and Counseling. 2005;57(2):153-7.

[46] Soundy A, Smith B, Dawes H, Pall H, Gimbrere K, Ramsay J. Patient's expression of hope and illness narratives in three neurological conditions: a meta-ethnography. Health Psychology Review. 2013;7(2):177-201.

[47] Bachmann C, Abramovitch H, Barbu CG, Cavaco AM, Elorza RD, Haak R, et al. A European consensus on learning objectives for a core communication curriculum in health care professions. Patient Education and Counseling. 2013;93(1):18-26.

[48] Légaré F, Ratté S, Gravel K, Graham ID. Barriers and facilitators to implementing shared decision-making in clinical practice: update of a systematic review of health professionals' perceptions. Patient Education and Counseling. 2008;73(3):526-35.

[49] West E, Barron DN, Reeves R. Overcoming the barriers to patient-centred care: time, tools and training. Journal of Clinical Nursing. 2005;14:435-43.

[50] Ford S, Schofield T, Hope T. Barriers to the evidence-based patient choice (EBPC) consultation. Patient Education and Counseling 2002;47:179-85.

[51] Williams C, Cantillon P, Cochrane M. The doctor-patient relationship: from undergraduate assumptions to pre-registration reality. Medical Education. 2001;35:743-7.

[52] Glenton C. Developing patient-centred information for back pain sufferers. Health Expectations. 2002;5:319-29.

[53] Esmaeili M, Cheraghi M, Salsali M. Barriers to patient-centered care: a thematic analysis study. International Journal of Nursing Knowledge. 2014;25(1):2-8.

[54] Lamb B, Taylor C, Lamb J, Strickland S, Vincent C, Green J, et al. Facilitators and barriers to teamworking and patient centeredness in multidisciplinary cancer teams: findings of a national study. Annals of Surgical Oncology. 2013;20:1408-16.

[55] Wittenberg-Lyles E, Goldsmith J, Ferrell B. Oncology nurse communication barriers to patient-centered care. Clinical Journal of Oncology Nursing. 2013;17(2):152-8.

[56] Yam B, Rossiter J. Caring in nursing: perceptions of Hong Kong nurses. Journal of Clinical Nursing. 2000;9(2):293-302.

[57] Kruijver I, Kerkstra A, Bensing J, van de Wiel H. Communication skills of nurses during interactions with simulated cancer patients. Journal of Advanced Nursing. 2001; 34(6):772-9.

[58] Jallinoja P, Absetz P, Kuronen R, Nissinen A, Talja M, Uutela A, et al. The dilemma of patient responsibility for lifestyle change: perceptions among primary care physicians and nurses. Scandinavian Journal of Primary Health Care. 2007;25(4):244–9.

[59] Chant S, Jenkinson T, Randle J, Russell G. Communication skills: some problems in nursing education and practice. Journal of Clinical Nursing. 2002;11:12-21.

[60] Haidet P, Dains J, Paterniti D, Hechtel L, Chang T, Tseng E, et al. Medical student attitudes toward the doctor-patient relationship. Medical Education 2002;36:568-74.

[61] Skaalvik M, Normann H, Henriksen N. Student experiences in learning person-centred care of patients with Alzheimer's disease as perceived by nursing students and supervising nurses. Journal of Clinical Nursing. 2010;19(17–18):2639-48.

[62] Suikkala A, Leino-Kilpi H. Nursing student-patient relationship: experiences of students and patients. Nurse Education Today. 2005;25(5):344-54.

[63] Tuohy D. Student nurse-older person communication. Nurse Education Today. 2003; 23(1):19-26.

[64] Kotecki C. Baccalaureate nursing students' communication process in the clinical setting. Journal of Nursing Education. 2002;41:61-8.

[65] Hjorleifsdottir E, Carter D. Communicating with terminally ill cancer patients and their families. Nurse Education Today. 2000;20(6):646-53.

[66] McCarthy B, O'Donovan M, Twomey A. Person-centred communication: design, implementation and evaluation of a communication skills module for undergraduate nursing students—an Irish context. Contemporary Nurse. 2008;27(2):207-22.

[67] Girdley D, Johnsen C, Kwekkeboom K. Facilitating a culture of safety and patient-centered care through use of a clinical assessment tool in undergraduate nursing education. Journal of Nursing Education. 2009;48(12):702-5.

[68] McKeon L, Norris T, Cardell B, Britt T. Developing patient-centered care competencies among prelicensure nursing students using simulation. Journal of Nursing Education. 2009;48(12):711-5.

[69] McKonkey R, Morris I, Purcell M. Communications between staff and adults with intellectual disabilities in naturally occurring settings. Journal of Intellectual Disability Research. 1999;43(3):194-205.

[70] Alasad J, Ahmad M. Communication with critically ill patients. Journal of Advanced Nursing. 2005;50(4):356-62.

[71] Hemsley B, Sigaffos J, Balandin S, Forbes R, Taylor C, Green V, et al. Nursing the patient with severe communication impairment. Journal of Advanced Nursing. 2001;35(6):827-35.

[72] Bastiaens H, Van Royen P, Pavlic D, Raposo V, Baker R. Older people's preferences for involvement in their own care: a qualitative study in primary health care in 11 European countries. Patient Education and Counseling. 2007;68(1):33-42.

[73] Curtis-Tyler K. Levers and barriers to patient-centred care with children: findings from a synthesis of studies of the experiences of children living with type 1 diabetes or asthma. Child: Care, Health and Development 2010;37(4):540-50.

[74] Windover AK, Boissy A, Rice TW, Gilligan T, Velez VJ, Merlino J. The REDE model of healthcare communication: optimizing relationship as a therapeutic agent. Journal of Patient Experience. 2014;1(1):8-13.

[75] Rider EA, Hinrichs MM, Lown BA. A model for communication skills assessment across the undergraduate curriculum. Medical Teacher. 2006;28(5):e127-34.

[76] Kurtz SM, Silverman JD, Draper J. Teaching and learning communication skills in medicine. 2nd ed. Oxford, UK: Radcliffe Medical Press; 2004.

[77] Frankel RM, Stein T. Getting the most out of the clinical encounter: the four habits model. Journal of Medical Practice Management. 2001;16(4):184-91.

[78] Baile W, Walters R. Challenging emotional conversations with patients and families: a guide to forming a therapeutic alliance with patients and families. wwwmdanderson-org/icare: Texas:The University of Texas MD Anderson Cancer Center; 2012.

[79] Bergin F. Successful presentations. Englewood Cliffs, NJ: Prentice Hall; 1995.

[80] Thompson BM, Teal CR, Scoot DM, Manning SN, Greenfiedl E, Shada R, et al. Following the clues: teaching medical students to explore patients' context. Patient Education and Counseling. 2010;80(3):345-50.

[81] Bleiker J, Knapp K, Frampton I. Teaching patient care to students: a blended learning approach in radiography education. Radiography 2011; 17(3): 235–40.

[82] Herxheimer A, McPherson A, Miller R, Shepperd S, Yaphe J, Ziebland S. Database of patients' experiences (DIPEx): a multi-media approach to sharing experiences and information. The Lancet. 2000;355(9214):1540-3.

[83] Maguire P, Pitceathly C. Key communication skills and how to acquire them. British Medical Journal. 2002;325(7366):697-700.

Chapter 4

Updated Landscape of the Tumor Microenvironment and Targeting Strategies in an Era of Precision Medicine

Yu Sun and Paul Chiao

Additional information is available at the end of the chapter

http://dx.doi.org/10.5772/66575

Abstract

Despite successive advances in clinical diagnosis and therapeutic intervention, cancer-associated morbidity and mortality keeps up with escalating cost to human society. Clinicians are confronted with an unprecedented challenge in curing cancers with *de novo* or acquired resistance. Failure to achieve effective and long-lasting treatment effects arises from the complexity of malignancies, particularly when plasticity of cancer cells is coupled with survival adaptability conferred by the pathologically co-opted stroma in the tumor microenvironment (TME). Targeting immune checkpoints, such as programmed cell death 1 (PD-1), programmed cell death ligand 1 (PD-L1) and cytotoxic T lymphocyte antigen 4 (CTLA4), provide significant benefit in multiple tumor types and produce substantial anticancer responses. Tissue resident stromal cells, although damaged together with cancer cells upon cytotoxic treatments, represent an ever-replenishing source that contributes to tumor restoration from residual cancer cells in the post-therapy stage. The TME displays a continually changing landscape, generating significant impacts on treatment outcome in clinics. Moving forward, implementing patient-specific analysis in clinical oncology with TME-oriented agents will significantly improve the specificity and efficacy of targeted therapies, thereby accelerating the translation of novel conceptions and groundbreaking discoveries in the TME biology through multiple bench-to-bed pipelines in current settings of precision cancer medicine.

Keywords: tumor microenvironment, cancer treatment, secretory phenotype, acquired resistance, precision medicine

1. Introduction

Tumor development implicates the coevolution of transformed cells and the surrounding TME. In solid organs, the TME comprises extracellular matrix, neovasculature and multiple stromal cell types, conferring neoplastic cells multiple capabilities including sustained growth, elevated migration, accelerated invasion, promoted drug resistance and more importantly, enhanced metastasis [1]. In contrast to cancer cells, stromal components in the TME are generally stable in genetics and represent a potentially ideal target for therapeutic intervention.

There is accelerated progress in both the design and application of anticancer therapies. However, to date, most clinical regimens including chemotherapy, radiation and targeted therapy fail to cure patients, even with the integration of cutting-edge techniques and facilities. The case is, cancers that show overt initial responses to treatments frequently relapse as resistant malignancies, and pathological relapse remains as a major challenge in clinical oncology. Tumor outgrowth and disease exacerbation relies on not only genetic modifications in somatic cells but also fitness advantages of such mutations provide within the TME. It is increasingly evident that heterologous cell lineages within the TME actively alter therapeutic response and shape cancer resistance [2]. The distinct TME attributes within a given tumor select for mutations that allow survival, expansion and repopulation of cancer cells, while significantly creating tumor heterogeneity. Such a plasticity promotes the development of drug resistance through several mechanisms, including mutations of the target genes, reactivation of the targeted pathways, and cancer cross talk with the surrounding TME, with the latter largely overlooked in the past decades [3]. Besides, mounting data support that stromal cells, either naïve or therapeutically damaged, can produce and secrete a large group of soluble factors into the TME milieu, which act as critical signals delivered in a paracrine fashion and dramatically confer therapeutic resistance on cancer cells. Therefore, the TME is biologically active in the course of disease progression and exerts pathological impacts in a spatiotemporally volatile manner, underscoring the necessity of considering the TME as a dynamic entity in designing novel agents and developing therapeutic strategies. In this chapter, we propose to offer a body of essential information that delivers an updated account of the newly emerging TME biology, provide a significant guide to the most recent literature, and envision prospects for future research in basic, translational and clinical medicine.

2. Main body

2.1. Pathological characteristics of the TME

In the microenvironment of healthy tissues, the stroma functions as a physical barrier against tumorigenesis. Nevertheless, cells transformed by intrinsic or extrinsic events can make major changes that stimulate the adjacent microenvironment to support disease progression. Such changes include remodeling of extracellular matrix (ECM), recruitment of fibroblasts, chemoattraction of immune cells, migration of neuroendocrine cells and networking of endothelial cells (vascularization). How do the genetic and/or epigenetic variations present within cancer cells generate a phenotypically complicated TME, which further exert profound influences on tumor development? The differences in selective pressures of *in vivo* conditions, such as local acidity, intermittent hypoxia and growth factor production within a tumor can actively shape the pathway of disease progression. Besides all the autonomous factors generated by the tumor itself, distinct environmental landscapes within the tumor foci select for mutations that engender increased malignancy, foster tumor heterogeneity and enhance therapeutic resistance, all factors closely correlated with decreased treatment efficacy and increased clinical failure.

As cancer cells expand at a given site and generate early insults that form the initial tumor niches, host-resident benign cell types coevolve with the neoplastic cells in the same tissue, both populations are continuously engaged in aging-related pathologies (**Figure 1**).

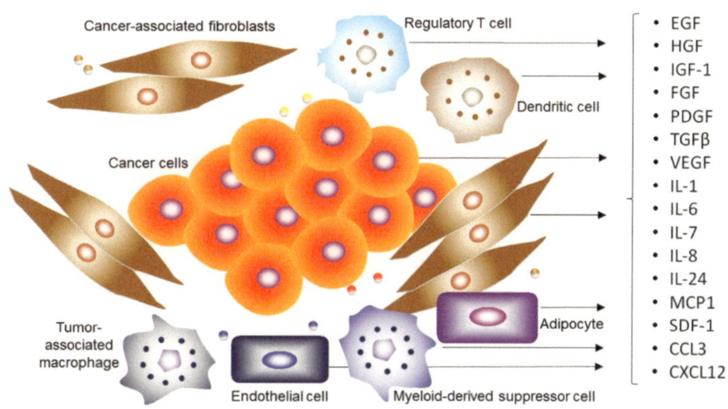

Figure 1. Schematic outline of cell type components within a typical TME. Although intercellular interactions confer various malignant potentials on cancer cells in the tumor foci, soluble factors released from cell subpopulations can actively suppress the local immune/inflammatory activities, thereby creating an inhibitory and hostile environmental niche for infiltrating cells recruited into the tumor from other sites. EGF, epidermal growth factor; HGF, hepatocyte growth factor; IGF-1, insulin-like growth factor-1; FGF, fibroblast growth factor; PDGF, platelet-derived growth factor; TGF-β, tumor growth factor-β; VEGF, vascular endothelial growth factor; IL, interleukin; MCP-1, monocytic chemotactic protein 1; SDF-1, stroma-derived factor 1; CCL3, chemokine C-C motif ligand 1; CXCL12, chemokine C-X-C motif 12.

2.1.1. Cancer-associated fibroblasts

Fibroblasts represent an abundant and predominant cell type that maintains the structural framework in the connective tissue of solid organs. Normal fibroblasts typically suppress tumor formation; however, cancer-associated fibroblasts (CAFs), to the contrary, mainly promote tumorigenesis and facilitate metastasis. Compared with their normal counterparts, CAFs exhibit increased proliferation, enhanced ECM production, accumulated basement membrane deposition, strengthened cytokine synthesis and secretion including hepatocyte growth factor (HGF), multiple interleukins (ILs), platelet-derived growth factor (PDGF), stromal cell-derived factor 1 (SDF1), tumor growth factor-β (TGF-β) and vascular endothelial growth factor (VEGF) [4]. Alternatively, other mesenchyme-derived cell types, such as adipocytes, can also contribute to tumor growth and disease progression. For instance, adiponectin from the differentiated adipocytes increases VEGF-A expression in human chondrosarcoma cells through adiponectin receptor (AdipoR), hypoxia-inducible factor-1α (HIF)-1α, phosphoinositide 3 kinase (PI3K), Akt and mammalian target of rapamycin (mTOR) signaling cascades [5].

There are debates on the origin of CAFs during cancer progression. Some data suggest that CAFs are derived from the endothelial-to-mesenchymal transition, whereas other studies support that epithelial-to-mesenchymal transition (EMT) is responsible for CAF production [6, 7].

CAFs accumulated in the TME are subject to activation by cytokines and growth factors present in the nearby niches, such as fibroblast growth factor (FGF), monocyte chemotactic protein 1 (MCP1), PDGF, TGF-β and secreted proteases [8, 9]. Once activated, CAFs release pro-inflammatory factors to activate the nuclear factor (NF)-KB signaling in transformed cells, a typical cell-cell cross talk that significantly promotes tumorigenesis [10]. In addition, CAFs in the mammary TME select for bone-specific metastatic traits in primary tumor cells, partially based on the mutual interaction between Src^+ breast cancer cells and CAFs that produce chemokine C-X-C motif ligand 12 (CXCL12) and insulin-like growth factor 1 (IGF1) [11]. A recent study suggested that circulating CAFs (cCAFs) with co-expressed fibroblast-associated protein (FAP) and α-smooth muscle actin (α-SMA) are distinguishable in the peripheral blood of patients with metastatic breast cancer. Furthermore, both cCAFs and circulating tumor cells (CTCs) are of significantly higher number in the metastatic group than in the localized breast cancer group, implying that cCAFs may complement CTCs as a clinically specific biomarker in metastatic breast cancer [12]. This also consolidates that functional roles of CAFs in tumor progression involve malignant activities not only in the primary foci but also in the systemic delivery of cancer cells of high metastatic potential to colonize in a foreign microenvironments, further supporting the interactions between cancer and TME in both the local and distant niches.

2.1.2. Neovasculature

Development of the tumor-associated vascular network is dynamic and dramatically influences tumor behaviors. Starting from regional angiogenesis, vascular networks are strengthened by co-opting mature vessels within the tissue, recruiting endothelial precursors from bone marrow. Specifically, neovascularization involves degradation and reconstruction of existing vascular basement membranes in a tissue-specific manner, as it evidenced by the fact that concurrent targeting of VEGF and Angiopoietin-2 (Ang2) potentiates the effectiveness of VEGF inhibition and prevents basement membrane destruction [13]. It is likely that newly co-opted vessels sustain certain properties of the original tissue, which exerts critical influences on the resulting vascular network.

However, deficient tumor vasculature such as unbalanced vessel development results in formation of hypoxic microenvironments with limited nutrient supplementation. Spatial interval from vascular beds to tumor foci creates a local gradient, a crucial factor for the distribution of anticancer agents within a given tumor tissue. In clinics, angiogenesis is assessed by microvessel density (MVD), an important prognostic factor for clinical outcomes of multiple tumor types. In prostate cancer, CD105-MVD reflects the angiogenic conditions in patients treated with neoadjuvant hormonal therapy (NHT) and acts as an emerging independent predictor of biochemical recurrence in prostate cancer patients after radical prostatectomy with NHT [14]. In addition, upregulation of pro-angiogenic ligand VEGFA is associated with a worse prognosis in metastatic colorectal, lung and renal cell cancers. For example, high VEGF expression was subsequently correlated with a short overall survival rate for colorectal cancer patients exhibiting lymph node metastasis [15].

2.1.3. Immune system

Upon disease progression, both the innate and adaptive immune systems are implicated in tumor-associated activities. Despite the ability of the immune system to mount antitumor responses, immune suppression mechanisms, however, often prevent such a process. Particularly, T-cell activation engages both positive and negative checkpoint signals to finely tune responses to avoid overt damage and autoimmunity. Particularly, cancer immunoediting is a process by which the immune system can paradoxically restrain or facilitate cancer progression [16]. The interaction between tumor and immune system is now regarded as a crucial factor relevant for the clinical management of cancer patients [17].

2.1.3.1. Checkpoint-associated immunosuppression

Blockade of immune checkpoints including cytotoxic T lymphocyte antigen 4 (CTLA4), programmed cell death 1 (PD-1) and programmed cell death ligand 1 (PD-L1) has achieved significant benefits in multiple cancer types by minimizing inhibitory signals while amplifying effective antitumor responses. Anti-CTLA4, PD-1 or PD-L1 administration as mono-immunotherapy have demonstrated clinical activity in more than 15 cancer types, including bladder carcinoma, Hodgkin lymphoma, melanoma, non-small cell lung carcinoma (NSCLC) and renal cell carcinoma (RCC) [18]. Although immune-based regimens for cancer treatment are expected to increase substantially within the next years, combinatorial inhibition of PD-1 and CTLA4 holds the potential to further enhance antitumor efficacy. Clinical efficacy of the combination of ipilimumab and nivolumab in the setting of malignant melanoma at advanced stage is recently witnessed, and successfully passed approval by the FDA for the treatment of patients with unresectable or metastatic melanoma harboring wild-type $BRAF^{V600}$ [19].

Thus, clinical data support that antitumor immunity is operative even in the most advanced cancer stages, and multiple immunosuppressive pathways are active in the TME which need to be co-targeted to release the full effector function of tumor-associated immune cells [20]. In fact, diverse additional immunomodulatory pathways and suppressive factors produced or secreted by stromal cells in the TME can be exploited as useful targets for immune checkpoint targeting [21]. However, some critical questions still remain open. For example, which combinations should move toward practical development? What type of patients will benefit most from such therapies? Systematic consideration of these issues by determining the leading drug targets expressed by cancer cells will allow substantial enhancement of the immune responses to eradicate the disease.

Immunological pathway	Examples in clinical trials	Most advanced stage of clinical development
CTLA4	Ipilimumab	FDA approved
	Tremelimumab	Phase III
PD1-PDL1	Pembrolizumab (PD1)	FDA approved
	Nivolumab (PD1)	FDA approved
	Atezolizumab (formerly MPDL3280A) (PDL1)	Phase III
	MEDI4736 (PDL1)	Phase III
	Avelumab (PDL1)	Phase I
	PDR001 (PD1)	Phase I
TNF and TNFR superfamilies		
4-1BB–4-1BB ligand	Urelumab, PF-05082566	Phase II
OX40–OX40 ligand	MEDI6469	Phase II
GITR	TRX518	Phase I
CD27	Varlilumab	Phase II
TNFRSF25–TL1A	–	Preclinical
CD40–CD40 ligand	CP-870893	Phase I
HVEM–LIGHT–LTA	–	Preclinical
HVEM–BTLA–CD160	–	Preclinical
IGSF		
LAG3	BMS-986016	Phase I
TIM3		Preclinical
Siglecs		Preclinical
B7 and CD28-related proteins		
ICOS–ICOS ligand	–	Preclinical
B7-H3	MGA271	Phase I
B7-H4	–	Preclinical
VISTA	–	Preclinical
HHLA2–TMIGD2	–	Preclinical
Butyrophilins, including BTNL2	–	Preclinical
CD244–CD48	–	Preclinical
TIGIT and PVR family members	–	Preclinical
Natural killer cell targets		
KIRs	Lirilumab	Phase II
ILTs and LIRs	–	Preclinical

NKG2D and NKG2A	IPH2201	Phase I
MICA and MICB	–	Preclinical
CD244	–	Preclinical
Suppressive myeloid cells		
CSF1R	Emactuzumab	Phase I
Soluble mediators		
IDO	INCB024360	Phase II
TGF-β	Galunisertib	Phase I
Adenosine–CD39–CD73	–	Preclinical
CXCR4–CXCL12	Ulocuplumab (BMS-936564), BKT140 (BL-8040), Plerixafor	Phase I/II*
Other		
Phosphatidylserine	Bavituximab	Phase II/III
SIRPA–CD47	CC-90002	Phase I
VEGF	Bevacizumab	FDA approved
Neuropilin	MNRP1685A	Phase I

BTLA, B and T lymphocyte attenuator; BTNL2, butyrophilin-like protein 2; CSF1R, macrophage colony-stimulating factor receptor 1; CTLA4, cytotoxic T lymphocyte antigen 4; CXCL12, chemokine (C-X-C motif) ligand 12; CXCR4, C-X-C chemokine receptor type 4; GITR, glucocorticoid-induced tumor necrosis factor receptor (TNFR)-related protein; HHLA2, HERV-H LTR-associating protein 2; HVEM, herpes virus entry mediator; ICOS, inducible T cell co-stimulator; IDO, indoleamine 2,3-dioxygenase; IGSF, immunoglobulin superfamily; ILT, immunoglobulin-like transcript; KIR, killer inhibitory immunoglobulin-like receptor; LAG3, lymphocyte activation gene 3 protein; LIR, leukocyte immunoglobulin-like; LTA, lymphotoxin-α; MIC, MHC class I polypeptide-related sequence; PD1, programmed cell death protein 1; PDL1, programmed cell death 1 ligand 1; PVR, poliovirus receptor; SIRPA, signal-regulatory protein-alpha; TGF-β, transforming growth factor-β; TIGIT, T cell immunoreceptor with immunoglobulin and ITIM domains; TIM3, T cell immunoglobulin mucin 3; TL1A, TNF-like ligand 1A; TMIGD2, transmembrane and immunoglobulin domain-containing protein 2; TNFRSF25, TNFR superfamily member 25; TNFR, TNF receptor; VEGF, vascular endothelial growth factor; VISTA, V-domain immunoglobulin suppressor of T cell activation.

*Plerixafor (Mozobil; Genzyme/Sanofi) is approved by the US Food and Drug Administration not as an antitumor therapy but as a bone marrow mobilizing agent for bone marrow transplantation including autologous cases. However, it is currently in clinical trials of chronic lymphocytic leukemia, multiple myeloma and non-Hodgkin''s lymphoma patients.

Contents of Table 1 adapted from Mahoney et al. [25] with permission from Nature Reviews Drug Discovery, copyright 2015.

Table 1. Representative immunotherapeutic targets currently in clinical or preclinical pipelines.

Concurrent inhibition of PD-1 and CTLA4 significantly increases response rate in melanoma patients and is now in Phase III trials in multiple cancer types [19, 22]. Since immunosuppression is dominant, it makes sense that a standard immunotherapy begins with immune checkpoint blockade instead of a direct immune stimulation. Release from immunosuppression will allow for combination with multiple immunotherapies that eventually activate the immune response. Results from the Phase I trial of synergistic CTLA4 and PD-1 blockade suggest that such a combination is clinically effective, but highly toxic to patients [19]. In this case, alternative combinations with the anti–PD-1 pathway backbone will likely produce better response in cancer clinics with fewer side effects. A group of immunological pathway candidates for combinatorial inhibition of the immune checkpoint is in various stages of clinical trials (**Table 1**). The corresponding agents are designed to directly stimulate cytotoxic T cells, block immunosuppressive factors, inhibit regulatory T cells (Treg) functions, interfere with the natural killer cell inhibitory activities or abolish the effects of soluble factors produced by stromal cells.

2.1.3.1.1. Tumor-associated macrophages (TAMs)

In solid tumors, TAMs compose 5–40% of the tumor mass and are usually correlated with poor prognosis. Distinct from M1-macrophages, the immune cell subpopulation of pro-inflammatory and anti-cancer properties, M2-macrophages are immunosuppressive, contributing to the matrix-remodeling and favor tumor progression [23]. TAMs are either tissue-resident or derived from peripheral sites including the bone marrow (BM) and spleen. Increasing lines of evidence suggest an active role for TAMs in supporting multiple malignant behaviors such as invasiveness at the leading edge of tumors. Particularly, studies have demonstrated that TAMs promote cancer cell invasion through a paracrine signaling loop involving tumor-associated granulocyte macrophage colony stimulating factor (GM-CSF) and macrophage-derived epidermal growth factor (EGF) in breast cancer and glioma [24, 25]. Additionally, the close vicinity of cancer cells in epithelial-mesenchymal transition (EMT) and TAMs at the invasive tumor front implies that these two cell type may mutually interact with each other. Beyond the leading edge, TAMs represent a major source of proteases including cysteine cathepsins, which promote tumor progression and therapeutic resistance in multiple cancer types [26].

However, it remains so far unclear how macrophages switch from tumor suppressing to tumor promoting upon disease progression. It is likely that environmental factors such as tumor hypoxia are involved in such a transition. Specifically, TAMs accumulate at sites of hypoxia in growing tumors, and their recruitment is mediated by macrophage chemoattractants such as endothelin-2 and VEGF [27]. Recent data further suggest that coexistence of hypoxia and free fatty acids (FFAs) exacerbates macrophage-mediated inflammation [28]. As noteworthy, TAM accumulation in these regions enhances angiogenesis and subsequent acquisition of invasive phenotype, supporting that the initial hypoxic response in growing tumors may induce a phenotypic switch of macrophages, which is correlated with their changed polarization [29].

2.1.3.1.2. Myeloid-derived suppressor cells (MDSCs) and Treg cells

In a typical TME, immunosuppressive effects may also be exerted by myeloid-derived suppressor cells (MDSCs), which result from aberrant myelopoiesis that occurs in developing tumors [30]. Functionally identified as an immunosuppressive subpopulation, MDSCs are immature myeloid cells that sustain normal tissue homeostasis upon stimulation of the host by various systemic insults such as viral infection and traumatic stress [31]. However, MDSCs dramatically promote tumor growth by supporting angiogenesis, cancer cell survival, tumor metastases and pre-metastatic niche formation [32]. In particular, the process of tumorigenesis can mobilize MDSCs which subsequently infiltrate developing tumors and promote local vascularization and disrupt routine immunosurveillance, including dendritic cell (DC) antigen presentation, M1 macrophage polarization, T cell activation and natural killer (NK) cell cytotoxicity blockade [33]. Depletion of MDSCs in animal models with neutralizing antibodies markedly reduced metastasis, further consolidating that MDSCs promote tumor progression [31]. Furthermore, cancer patients display elevated numbers of peripheral MDSCs, which is positively associated with the disease aggravation extent and therapeutic failure rate [34]. Interestingly, monocytic MDSCs can be reprogrammed to exhibit an antitumorigenic phenotype upon bacteria-elicited activation of the immune system in animal models [35]. In such a case, increased T helper type 1 (T_H1) cytokines, decreased T cell-inhibitory factors and differentiation of MDSCs toward M1-like macrophages were observed, suggesting that immunotherapies are able to subvert autonomous responses of MDSCs to extrinsic stimuli to maintain homeostasis, an exploitable aspect of such an immune cell subgroup in cancer treatment.

Phenotypically, Treg cells represent another TME cell type with multiple immune modulatory functions in human cancer patients. As an essential part of the normal tissue under physiological conditions, Treg cells control the proliferation and activation of adaptive immune system including T and B cells, thus having a critical role in homeostasis maintenance. However, Treg cells can generate diverse effects on tumorigenesis. For example, increased numbers of Treg cells are correlated with poor survival of several pathologies including lung, colorectal and estrogen receptor (ER)-negative breast cancer; however, their role on prostate and ER-positive breast tumor development remains uncertain [36]. Similar to MDSCs, Treg cells prevent tumor-associated antigen presentation and suppress cytotoxic T cell function by blocking the release of cytolytic granules [37].

In nature, tumor-associated Treg cells have heterogeneous phenotypes, and they may accumulate through various mechanisms including peripheral recruitment, TME-based proliferation or progenitor-initiated differentiation upon stimulation by tumor-secreted factors [38]. Thus, CD25 antibody-involved Treg-targeting or other treatment regimens may promote immunotherapy responses, like agents designed for MDSCs [39].

2.1.3.1.3. Other stromal cell types implicated in tumor progression

Several stromal cell types recently emerged with the potential to generate remarkable influences on human cancer. Particularly, adipocytes and their progenitors in obese populations promote tumorigenesis across a handful of obesity-related cancer types [40, 41]. Adipocytes cause the enrichment of prostate cancer stem cells (CSCs) through a distinct cycle of autocrine amplification, suggesting a novel mechanism underlying the mutual interaction between adipocytes and prostate CSCs [42]. Moreover, adipose cells can be recruited to growing tumor foci, differentiating into pericytes and incorporating into vessel walls [43]. In both the basement membrane (BM) and local environment of solid tumors, atypical stem-promoting functions of nerves can enhance the aggressiveness of cancer cells, including those in gastrointestinal, pancreatic and prostate tumors [44–46]. Furthermore, inflammation associated with the gut microbiome is considered as one of the major contributing factor of colorectal cancer outcomes. The US National Institutes of Health has recently launched an initiation to thorough study the human microbiome in various anatomical sites including the gut [47]. Targeting agents with anti-inflammatory (such as aspirin) or antimicrobial efficacy can prevent colorectal cancer tumorigenesis, thereby elongating patient survival [48]. Given the emergence of non-classical stromal cell types in solid tumors, creative combination anticancer therapies are being continually developed in the industrial pipelines and will show promising benefits in mitigating disease progression.

2.1.4. Tumor-associated exosomes

Diverse signaling activities within the TME involve autocrine and/or paracrine signaling loops of cytokines, chemokines and growth factors. Besides such a typical aspect, exosome-based shedding has recently emerged as an alternative modality of cell-cell communication. In particular, tumor-derived exosomes from the primary site reprogram the surrounding TME to form a pro-tumorigenic niche, orchestrating BM-derived progenitors to facilitate metastatic dissemination [49]. A recent study demonstrated that tumor-associated exosomes express unique integrins and determine organotropic metastasis through creating pre-metastatic niches via integrin-mediated fusion with organ-specific resident cells [50]. Aggressive melanoma-derived exosomes increase tumor metastasis rates and programs BMDCs at the pre-metastatic sites to form a proangiogenic phenotype [51]. More importantly, multiple stromal cell types can release exosomes, as exemplified by fibroblast-secreted exosomes which promote cell migration through WNT-PCP signaling in breast cancer [52]. In such a case, NK cell-derived exosomes from human blood harbor proteins to induce the tumor cytotoxicity and activate immune cells *ex vivo*. Conversely, new data demonstrated that endometrial cancer cells transmit small regulatory RNAs to endometrial fibroblasts through exosomes, suggesting a reciprocal mode of intercellular communication between cancer cells and related fibroblasts in human tumors [53]. Distinct prostate cancer (PCa) cell populations release exosomes that contain miRNAs to modify the local or pre-metastatic niche, and such miRNAs have different patterns between PCa bulk and CSCs exosomes that function collaboratively in tumor progression and metastasis [54]. The most abundant exosomes-related miRNAs thus can be regarded as potentially significant biomarkers and therapeutic targets in clinical oncology.

2.2. The therapeutically remodeled TME alters clinical outcome

Recent studies have recognized benign or noncancerous cells of the TME are major determinants of treatment efficacy in a large number of preclinical and clinical cases, an important mechanism of acquired resistance that is beyond the intrinsic characteristics of cancer cells but use to be masked by the *de novo* resistance of malignancies. Insightful appreciation of mechanisms involved in regulation of drug tolerance is crucial for improved cancer treatment. Specifically, host resident cells of the TME actively modulate tumor responses to chemotherapy and targeted therapies through production of secreted factors [55].

Neoadjuvant or conventional chemotherapy-induced DNA damage can cause WNT16B overexpression, a phenomenon found in the TME of prostate, breast and ovarian cancer patients. Upon genotoxic insults, NF-κB acts as a key signaling node that actively mediates WNT16B production. Cell-based experiments and tumor transplant models demonstrated the protective effect of fibroblast-derived WNT16B, indicating that WNT16B secreted by stroma attenuates cancer cell apoptosis induced by genotoxicity, and counteracts drug response through activation of a DNA damage secretory program (DDSP) [56–59] (**Figure 2**). The study presents new opportunities for future advanced treatments that rationally integrate agents to confine the TME activities. For instance, depleting stroma-derived WNT16B, which would specifically overcome such a "new" but not "minor" TME-associated resistance mechanism [57, 60]. As supporting evidence, CAFs are similarly enriched in colorectal cancer (CRC) during the post-therapy stage and display enhanced cytokine IL-17A, which helps maintain the tumor infiltrating cells (TICs) through activation of NF-κB signaling [61].

Besides overturning traditional law of nature that anticancer treatments mainly restrain cancer cells, the discovery raises the novel appreciation that genotoxic regimens including chemotherapy and radiation indeed activate the stroma to promote disease resistance, an important advancement corroborated by several other concurrent but mutually independent reports of breast cancer models that strongly imply DNA damage-elicited alterations of the TME as an pathological entity that eventually minimizes the overall therapeutic response [62, 63]. The BM is enriched with cells of varying progeny beyond myeloid cell populations that are mobilized and recruited to the TME in response to treatments. Importantly, BM-derived mesenchymal stem cells (BMMSCs) can secrete polyunsaturated fatty acids, chemoprotective factors that favor cancer cell survival [64]. Although the data showed that only the cisplatin-involving therapy can induce such a change, the TME-derived fatty acids eventually conferred resistance to multiple agents even at a systemic level. Alternatively, therapeutic evasion by cancer propagating cells (CPC) represents a major obstacle in leukemia clinics. Recent data showed that the BM niche is created by acute lymphoblastic leukemia (ALL) cells following cytarabine and daunorubicin treatment [65]. Mesenchymal cells recruited by leukemia cell-derived CCL3 can build a therapy-induced shelter and evolve from Nestin+ cells to a smooth muscle actin (a-SMA)+ cells under TGF-β influence, ultimately developing into fiber residues. Formation of such an early protective niche significantly contributes to the failure of therapeutic intervention by preventing complete remission.

Cocultured fibroblasts regulate the *in vitro* sensitivity of head and neck squamous cell carcinoma (HNSCC) to epithelial growth factor receptor (EGFR) antibodies or matrix metalloproteinase (MMP) inhibitors [66]. Furthermore, tumor-stroma cross talk plays a crucial role in the acquisition of lung cancer resistance to EGFR-tyrosine kinase inhibitors (TKIs) through activating the c-Met/PI3K/Akt pathway *in vitro* and *in vivo*, implying such an interaction may be therapeutically targeted for lung cancer patients with EGFR-activating mutations [67]. HGF represents one of the major stroma-released soluble regulators of lung cancer sensitivity, whereas gefitinib in synergy with anti-HGF antibody or the HGF antagonist NK4 showed decent efficacy in abolishing fibroblast-induced EGFR-TKI resistance. Similarly, co-inhibition of EGFR and c-Met signaling with a novel bi-specific EGFR/c-Met antibody effectively blocked malignant development including resistance additively compared with the single-agent treatments [68].

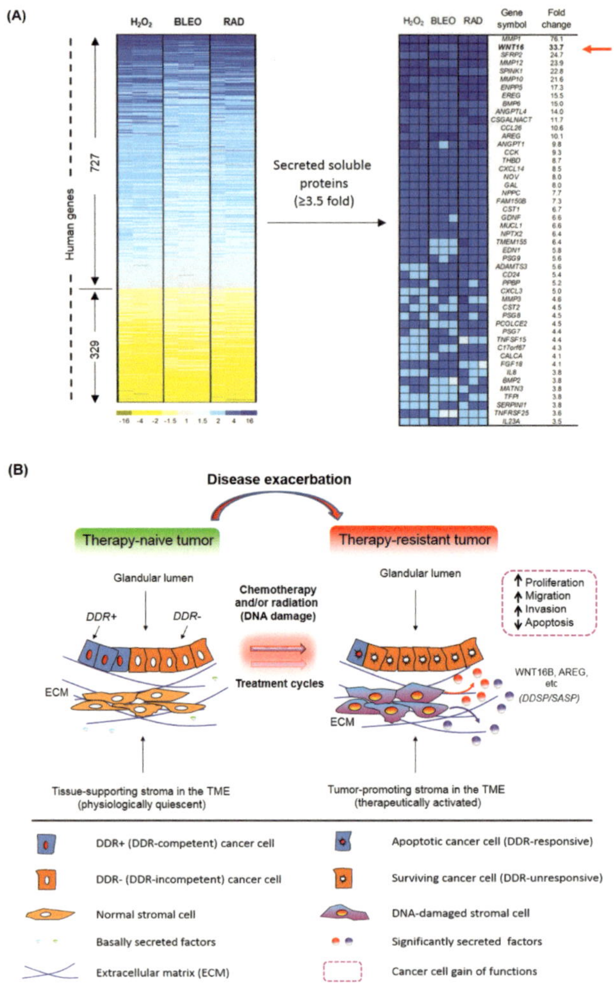

Figure 2. WNT16B is significantly produced upon genotoxic damage to human stromal cells and promotes therapeutic resistance to surviving cancer cells. (**A**) Genome-wide expression pattern of normal human primary prostate stromal cells. Heatmap depicts the relative mRNA abundance after exposure of cells to typical DNA damaging agents (H_2O_2, hydrogen peroxide; Bleo, bleomycin; Rad, ionizing radiation). (**B**) Top list of upregulated human genes annotated as extracellular or secreted factors, with average expression fold change ≥3.5 by comparison of post-treatment vs. pre-treatment samples. Note, WNT16B shows up among the overexpressed genes, with outstanding expression fold change. (**C**) Working model for cancer cell non-autonomous therapeutic resistance acquired from the TME upon genotoxic treatments including chemotherapy and radiation. Therapeutic agents cause apoptosis in subsets of cancer cells by eliciting a DNA damage response (DDR), while cancer cells with DDR deficiency (DDR-insensitive, or DDR-) may escape from such insults. Simultaneously, senescence is induced in stromal cells adjacent to epithelial cells surrounding the gland, with a secretory phenotype DDSP developed after DDR events. A persistently activated signaling network is triggered by the DNA strand breaks. The DDSP is usually characterized by a spectrum of autocrine- and paracrine-acting proteins. The soluble factors reinforce the senescent phenotype in damaged cells, enhance cancer cell repopulation, with increased occurrence of tumor relapse and distant metastasis. A handful of co-synthesized factors including WNT16B and SPINK1 holds the potential to serve as both a serum biomarker to determine treatment index and a therapeutic target to minimize the TME-conferred therapeutic resistance. DDR, DNA damage response; ECM, extracellular matrix; TME, tumor microenvironment. Color images of (**A**) adapted from Xu et al. with permission from Trends in Cancer, copyright 2016.

The development and maintenance of vasculature is regulated by diverse pathways, including those engaging proangiogenic factors produced by both the tumor and stroma [69]. Upon genotoxic treatments, stromal expression of VEGF and other angiogenic factors including angiopoietin 1 (ANGPT1) and angiopoietin-like 4 (ANGPTL4) is enhanced, potentially contributing to vasculature development within the therapeutically damaged TME [56, 70]. Expression of the secreted frizzled-related protein 2 (SFRP2), a typical modulator of Wnt signaling, is increased in the stroma damaged by the chemotherapeutic cycles [56]. Beyond holding the potential to promote angiogenesis via the calcineurin/NFAT signaling in a non-canonical Wnt pathway [71, 72], SFRP2 can interact directly with WNT16B to enhance its canonical activities, eventually generating a substantially strengthened malignant phenotype including remarkable drug resistance in prostate cancer [73]. Data from targeting angiopoietins (Ang1, Ang2, Ang4) which cause CAF accumulation and neoangiogenesis in the TME, and TEK (referring to Tie1/Tie2) receptors responsible for the maturation and plasticity of blood vessels, are recently reported [74, 75]. Inhibiting angiogenesis in patients to overcome one of the side effects caused by cytotoxic agents is thus a novel strategy to block neoplastic growth and deprive cancer of acquired resistance.

Increasing lines of evidence support that the TME is critical for the development of chemoresistance through multiple mechanisms including drug distribution regulation and inflammatory response control. Particularly, the infiltration of myeloid-derived cells is increased in human breast cancer post-chemotherapy, with the cellular composition as a strong clinical predictor of overall survival [63]. Furthermore, myeloid cell-derived MMP9 influences both vascular leakage and response to chemotherapeutic drugs including doxorubicin. Therefore, tumor response to classical chemotherapeutic agents can be improved by targeting the TME with chemicals or antibodies that modify MMP activity and/or chemokine signaling. In another perspective, cancer treatments currently applied as the mainstay of clinical oncology indeed represent a double-edged sword, which is frequently compromised in reality by a therapeutically remodeled TME. The structural change, and more importantly, the functional modification of such a TME, casts a critical step toward development of more advanced malignancies including but not limited to the phenotypic switch via EMT, generation of circulating tumor cells (CTCs), local invasion in primary foci and metastasis to distant organs [76].

2.3. Development of targeting strategies in precision medicine

While the functional constituents of the TME generate profound impacts on disease progression and minimize the efficacy of anticancer therapies, experimental data indicate that such alterations are indeed exploitable and can open new avenues to develop advanced strategies and design innovative cancer regimens.

To date, there are a few leading research groups that have made progress in the TME biology by generating relevant databases and presenting therapeutic opportunities to prevent TME-induced cancer resistance. First of all, cytokines, growth factors and survival-associated proteins released by the TME are straightforward and valid therapeutic targets. As an efficient growth stimulator, IL-6 enhances resistance by counteracting chemotherapy and hormone therapy of multiple myeloma; it is also a therapeutic target in Castleman's disease and several epithelial malignancies including mammary, breast ovarian, prostate cancers [77]. Recent data demonstrated that HGF is a critical TME determinant of resistance to BRAF inhibitors, setting the baseline for combinations of HGF-targeting monoclonal antibodies and RTK inhibitors that dampen the receptor c-Met activation [78, 79]. Identification of the distinct role of stroma-derived WNT16B in prostate cancer strongly supports translational studies in cancer therapy, as evidenced by the pilot preclinical trial integrating a monoclonal WNT16B antibody and routine chemotherapy to treat prostate tumors [73]. It is tempting to compare the efficacy of WNT16B-implicated pathway blockade and a wider suppression of the TME response to genotoxicity by inactivating the NF-κB complex. As the NF-κB activity differs between various stromal cell lineages upon therapeutic insults, it would be necessary to compare the effects of NF-κB suppression in individual TME-derived cell types. Nevertheless, there are caveats when selecting NF-κB as a general therapeutic target, although accumulating experimental data have established the NF-κB complex as a key regulator of inflammation and a driver of cancer progression. However, reverse but convincing data proved that activated NF-κB components enhance the sensitivity of cancer cells to chemicals that induce apoptosis and senescence, a special mechanism that controls tumorigenesis [80, 81]. As a supporting point, canonical NF-κB is found to be a Fas transcription activator, though the alternative NF-κB acts as a Fas transcription repressor [82]. In such a case, NF-κB promotes Fas-mediated cancer cell apoptosis, while suppression of NF-κB may abolish the Fas-initiated cell death and interfere with tumor regression achieved by the host immune system.

Strategies to inhibit the cancer resistance acquired from the TME in the course of either chemotherapy or targeted therapy have the value to improve overall therapeutic outcome. Generally, the TME exerts pathological influence on cancer cell survival as an early stage, while subsequent repopulation frequently occurs via the activation of signaling networks that elicit a typical secretory phenotype and/or tumor-stroma cross talk. To date, an array of agents are developed to minimize these activities, particularly small molecule inhibitors against key signal pathway nodes including the ATM/ATR-associated DDR repair machinery, p38MAPK cascade, mTOR subunits, JAK/STAT axis, NF-κB complex and CCAAT/enhancer binding protein (C/EBP) components. Alternatively, cytostatic antibodies with the ability to neutralize major soluble factors of significant roles in shaping advanced cancer phenotypes, such as those targeting MMPs, IL-6, IL-8, WNT16B, SFRP2, SPINK1 and AREG are also strong candidates that can be exploited to target the TME [57]. Fortunately, a handful of agents successfully acquired FDA approval for the systemic intervention of cancer patients while many others are in the industrial pipelines or clinical trials. As scientific acumen, an optimal therapeutic strategy is to consider the cancer a systemic disease at diagnosis and to pursue combinational therapy that incorporate cytotoxic agents and feasible cytostatic drugs either concurrently or sequentially, the latter actually more preferred [83]. Continued efforts in future will consolidate preclinical studies with novel therapeutics that deprive cancer of TME-conferred resistance, which is administered synergistically with cancer-targeting agents in pathological conditions that implicate a stress-responsive and functionally active TME.

Recently achieved in-depth profiling of cancer mutations by deep sequencing has enabled appreciation of the importance of tumor neoantigens in the immune surveillance of cancer, with the dream of "personalized immunotherapy" now realized. In particular, conceptual developments in cancer biology have caused a paradigm shift in the perspective we look at the TME when taking account of the immune system and its interaction with cancer. A simple but useful pragmatic framework allowing to stratify the TME into four classes according to the presence or absence of tumor-infiltrating lymphocytes (TILs) and PD-L1 expression was raised [84]. The proportion of tumors categorized as type I (~38%) and type II (~41%) by this framework is high in melanoma, and type I TME-harboring patients have the best prognosis and highest likelihood to respond to anti–PD-1/PD-L1 agents [85, 86]. Some malignancies such as prostate and pancreatic cancers, however, may not contain a high proportion of type I TME; in such a case, anti–PD-1/PD-L1 monotherapies are not expected to be highly effective [87]. Therefore, it is important to clarify which aspects of cancer immunity need to be targeted by novel immunotherapies, with the aim to provide benefit for patients with non-type I TME tumors. Different types of therapeutic interventions may need to be combined to generate a strong antitumor response, by effectively engaging immunity to suppress specific types of TME [17].

To treat various types of cancer-immune microenvironments, anti–PD-1 and anti–PD-L1 drugs will probably set the baseline of many future treatments for cancer, whereas the opportunities to combine these agents with surgery, radiation, immunogenic chemotherapy and targeted therapy and in class I tumors can be easily foreseen. The alternative strategy of chimeric antigen receptor T (CAR-T)-cell immunotherapy is essentially a combination treatment in nature. Providing earlier combination therapies to cancer patients, it is likely that approximately 50% or more of cancer types particularly some solid tumors such as melanoma and renal cell carcinoma are effectively prevented or controlled

3. Concluding remarks and future directions

Traditional anticancer treatments with cytotoxic drugs have generated limited promotion in the cure rates of various malignancies. Chemotherapy, radiation and targeted therapy, however, still have a large place in cancer clinics. Using novel approaches derived from the development of systems medicine, we will have a more thorough and accurate understanding of human cancer complexity and will be able to stratify patients appropriately. Personalized medicine has the potential to bring the best outcome for cancer patients, while healthcare costs should be made affordable and, most importantly, the combination therapies must be designed in a safe, rational, and effective way.

The fast moving research areas have undoubtedly set the stage for future investigation on interactions between cancer cells and the surrounding shelter, the TME. Development of methods for high content profiling of this complex biological landscape, and the other side, advancement of therapeutic strategies to overcome the pathological problem at a systemic level, thus turns out to be a very important task for prospective research and clinical practice.

Acknowledgements

The authors apologize to investigators whose work is not cited due to space limitations. They thank Dr. Peter Nelson (Fred Hutchinson Cancer Research Center, USA) and Dr. Judith Campisi (Buch Institute for Research on Aging, USA) for kindly providing fibroblast cell lines and conferring critical comments. This work is supported by a US DoD PCRP Idea Development Award (PC111703), National Natural Science Foundation of China (81472709) and the National 1000 Youth Elites Research Program of China to YS.

Abbreviations

ADCC	Antibody-dependent cellular cytotoxicity
AdipoR	Adiponectin receptor
ADP	Antibody-dependent phagocytosis
ALDH	Aldehyde dehydrogenase
ALL	Acute lymphoblastic leukemia
α-SMA	α-Smooth muscle actin
AML	Acute myeloid leukemia
ANGPTL4	Angiopoietin-like 4
ANGPT1	Angiopoietin 1
BM	Basement membrane or bone marrow
BMSC	Bone marrow stroma cell
CAF	Carcinoma-associated fibroblast
CAM-DR	Cell adhesion-mediated drug resistance
CAR-T	Chimeric antigen receptor T
cCAF	Circulating CAF
CCL2	Chemokine (C-C) ligand 2
CCL18	Chemokine (C–C) ligand 18
C/EBP	CCAAT/enhancer-binding protein
CLL	Chronic lymphocytic leukemia
CPC	Cancer-propagating cell
CSC	Cancer stem cell
CSF-1	Colony-stimulating factor 1
CTC	Circulating tumor cell
CTL	Cytotoxic T lymphocyte
CTLA4	Cytotoxic T lymphocyte antigen 4
CXCL12	Chemokine (C-X-C) ligand 12

http://dx.doi.org/10.5772/66575

CXCR4	Chemokine (C-X-C) ligand receptor 4
DC	Dendritic cell
DDR	DNA damage response
DDSP	DNA damage secretory program
ECM	Extracellular matrix
EGF	Epidermal growth factor
EMT	Epithelial-mesenchymal transition
ER	Estrogen receptor
ErbB2 (or Her2)	Human epidermal growth factor receptor 2
FAP	Fibroblast-activating protein or fibroblast-associated protein
FGF	Fibroblast growth factor
FSP1	Fibroblast-specific protein 1
GM-CSF	Granulocyte macrophage colony-stimulating factor
HGF	Hepatocyte growth factor
HIF1α	Hypoxia-inducible factor 1α
HNSCC	Head and neck squamous cell carcinoma
hTERT	Human telomerase reverse transcriptase
IGF-1	Insulin growth factor 1
IL	Interleukin
MAPK	Mitogen-activated protein kinase
MCP1	Monocyte chemotactic protein 1
MDR	Multiple drug resistance
MDSC	Myeloid-derived suppressor cell
MMP	Matrix metalloproteinase
MRD	Minimal residue disease
mTOR	Mammalian target of rapamycin
MVD	Microvessel density
NF-κB	Nuclear factor kappa-light-chain-enhancer of activated B cells
NHT	Neoadjuvant hormonal therapy
NK	Natural killer
NSCLC	Non-small cell lung cancer
PCa	Prostate cancer
PDGF	Platelet-derived growth factor
PD-1	Programmed cell death 1
PD-L1	Programmed cell death ligand 1
PI3K	Phosphoinositide 3 kinase

RCC	Renal cell carcinoma
RTK	Receptor tyrosine kinase
SCLC	Small-cell lung cancer
SDF-1	Stromal cell-derived growth factor 1
SFRP2	Secreted frizzled-related protein 2
TAM	Tumor-associated macrophage
TGF-β	Transforming growth factor-β
T_H1	T helper type 1
TIC	Tumor-infiltrating cell
TIL	Tumor-infiltrating lymphocyte
TKI	Tyrosine kinase inhibitor
TME	Tumor microenvironment
TNBC	Triple-negative breast cancer
TNF	Tumor necrosis factor
Treg	Regulatory T cell
uPAR	Urokinase plasminogen activator receptor
Vegf	Vascular endothelial growth factor

Author details

Yu Sun[1,2,3*] and Paul Chiao[1,4]

*Address all correspondence to: sunyu@sibs.ac.cn

1 Key Laboratory of Stem Cell Biology, Institute of Health Sciences, Shanghai Institutes for Biological Sciences, Chinese Academy of Sciences and Shanghai Jiaotong University School of Medicine, Shanghai, China

2 Collaborative Innovation Center of Systems Biomedicine, Shanghai Jiaotong University School of Medicine, Shanghai, China

3 Department of Medicine and VAPSHCS, University of Washington, Seattle, WA, USA

4 Department of Molecular and Cellular Oncology, The University of Texas MD Anderson Cancer Center, Houston, TX, USA

http://dx.doi.org/10.5772/66575

References

[1] Gu L, Mooney DJ. Biomaterials and emerging anticancer therapeutics: engineering the microenvironment. Nature Reviews Cancer. 2016;16:56–66.

[2] Junttila MR, de Sauvage FJ. Influence of tumour micro-environment heterogeneity on therapeutic response. Nature. 2013;501:346–354.

[3] Ramos P, Bentires-Alj M. Mechanism-based cancer therapy: resistance to therapy, therapy for resistance. Oncogene. 2015;34:3617–3626.

[4] Polanska UM, Orimo A. Carcinoma-associated fibroblasts: Non-neoplastic tumour-promoting mesenchymal cells. Journal of Cellular Physiology. 2013;228:1651–1657.

[5] Lee HP, Lin CY, Shih JS, Fong YC, Wang SW, Li TM, et al. Adiponectin promotes VEGF-A-dependent angiogenesis in human chondrosarcoma through PI3K, Akt, mTOR, and HIF-α pathway. Oncotarget. 2015;6:36746–36761.

[6] Zeisberg EM, Potenta S, Xie L, Zeisberg M, Kalluri R. Discovery of endothelial to mesenchymal transition as a source for carcinoma-associated fibroblasts. Cancer Research. 2007;67:10123–10128.

[7] Orr B, Riddick AC, Stewart GD, Anderson RA, Franco OE, Hayward SW, et al. Identification of stromally expressed molecules in the prostate by tag-profiling of cancer-associated fibroblasts, normal fibroblasts and fetal prostate. Oncogene. 2012;31:1130–1142.

[8] Dumont N, Liu B, Defilippis RA, Chang H, Rabban JT, Karnezis AN, et al. Breast fibroblasts modulate early dissemination, tumorigenesis, and metastasis through alteration of extracellular matrix characteristics. Neoplasia. 2013;15:249–262.

[9] Marsh T, Pietras K, McAllister SS. Fibroblasts as architects of cancer pathogenesis. BBA-Molecular Basis of Disease. 2013;1832:1070–1078.

[10] Erez N, Truitt M, Olson P, Arron ST, Hanahan D. Cancer-associated fibroblasts are activated in incipient neoplasia to orchestrate tumor-promoting inflammation in an NF-kappaB-dependent manner. Cancer Cell. 2010;17:135–147.

[11] Zhang XH, Jin X, Malladi S, Zou Y, Wen YH, Brogi E, et al. Selection of bone metastasis seeds by mesenchymal signals in the primary tumor stroma. Cell. 2013;154:1060–1073.

[12] Ao Z, Shah SH, Machlin LM, Parajuli R, Miller PC, Rawal S, et al. Identification of cancer-associated fibroblasts in circulating blood from patients with metastatic breast cancer. Cancer Research. 2015;75:4681–4687.

[13] Coutelle O, Schiffmann LM, Liwschitz M, Brunold M, Goede V, Hallek M, et al. Dual targeting of Angiopoetin-2 and VEGF potentiates effective vascular normalisation without inducing empty basement membrane sleeves in xenograft tumours. British Journal of Cancer. 2015;112:495–503.

[14] Miyata Y, Mitsunari K, Asai A, Takehara K, Mochizuki Y, Sakai H. Pathological significance and prognostic role of microvessel density, evaluated using CD31, CD34, and CD105 in prostate cancer patients after radical prostatectomy with neoadjuvant therapy. The Prostate. 2015;75:84–91.

[15] Kimura Y, Morohashi S, Yoshizawa T, Suzuki T, Morohashi H, Sakamoto Y, et al. Clinicopathological significance of vascular endothelial growth factor, thymidine phosphorylase and microvessel density in colorectal cancer. Molecular Medicine Reports. 2016;13:1551–1557.

[16] Teng MW, Galon J, Fridman WH, Smyth MJ. From mice to humans: developments in cancer immunoediting. The Journal of Clinical Investigation. 2015;125:3338–3346.

[17] Smyth MJ, Ngiow SF, Ribas A, Teng MW. Combination cancer immunotherapies tailored to the tumour microenvironment. Nature Reviews Clinical Oncology. 2016;13:143–158.

[18] Sharma P, Allison JP. The future of immune checkpoint therapy. Science. 2015;348:56–61.

[19] Wolchok JD, Kluger H, Callahan MK, Postow MA, Rizvi NA, Lesokhin AM, et al. Nivolumab plus ipilimumab in advanced melanoma. The New England Journal of Medicine. 2013;369:122–133.

[20] Melero I, Berman DM, Aznar MA, Korman AJ, Perez Gracia JL, Haanen J. Evolving synergistic combinations of targeted immunotherapies to combat cancer. Nature Reviews Cancer. 2015;15:457–472.

[21] Mahoney KM, Rennert PD, Freeman GJ. Combination cancer immunotherapy and new immunomodulatory targets. Nature Reviews Drug Discovery. 2015;14:561–584.

[22] Postow MA, Chesney J, Pavlick AC, Robert C, Grossmann K, McDermott D, et al. Nivolumab and ipilimumab versus ipilimumab in untreated melanoma. The New England Journal of Medicine. 2015;372:2006–2017.

[23] Sousa S, Brion R, Lintunen M, Kronqvist P, Sandholm J, Monkkonen J, et al. Human breast cancer cells educate macrophages toward the M2 activation status. Breast Cancer Research. 2015;17:101.

[24] Coniglio SJ, Eugenin E, Dobrenis K, Stanley ER, West BL, Symons MH, et al. Microglial stimulation of glioblastoma invasion involves epidermal growth factor receptor (EGFR) and colony stimulating factor 1 receptor (CSF-1R) signaling. Molecular Medicine. 2012;18:519–527.

[25] Su SC, Liu Q, Chen JQ, Chen JN, Chen F, He CH, et al. A positive feedback loop between mesenchymal-like cancer cells and macrophages is essential to breast cancer metastasis. Cancer Cell. 2014;25:605–620.

[26] Shree T. Macrophages and cathepsin proteases blunt chemotherapeutic response in breast cancer. Genes & Development. 2011;25:2465–2479.

[27] Lewis C, Murdoch C. Macrophage responses to hypoxia: implications for tumor progression and anti-cancer therapies. The American Journal of Pathology. 2005;167:627–635.

[28] Snodgrass RG, Boss M, Zezina E, Weigert A, Dehne N, Fleming I, et al. Hypoxia potentiates palmitate-induced pro-inflammatory activation of primary human macrophages. The Journal of Biological Chemistry. 2015;291:413–424.

[29] Escribese MM, Casas M, Corbi AL. Influence of low oxygen tensions on macrophage polarization. Immunobiology. 2012;217:1233–1240.

[30] Gabrilovich D, Nefedova Y. ROR1C regulates differentiation of myeloid-derived suppressor cells. Cancer Cell. 2015;28:147–149.

[31] Talmadge JE, Gabrilovich DI. History of myeloid-derived suppressor cells. Nature Reviews Cancer. 2013;13:739–752.

[32] Condamine T, Ramachandran I, Youn JI, Gabrilovich DI. Regulation of tumor metastasis by myeloid-derived suppressor cells. Annual Review of Medicine. 2015;66:97–110.

[33] Quail DF, Joyce JA. Microenvironmental regulation of tumor progression and metastasis. Nature Medicine. 2013;19:1423–1437.

[34] Arina A, Bronte V. Myeloid-derived suppressor cell impact on endogenous and adoptively transferred T cells. Current Opinion in Immunology. 2015;33:120–125.

[35] Shirota Y, Shirota H, Klinman DM. Intratumoral injection of CpG oligonucleotides induces the differentiation and reduces the immunosuppressive activity of myeloid-derived suppressor cells. The Journal of Immunology. 2012;188:1592–1599.

[36] Barth SD, Schulze JJ, Kuhn T, Raschke E, Husing A, Johnson T, et al. Treg-Mediated immune tolerance and the risk of solid cancers: findings from EPIC-Heidelberg. Journal of the National Cancer Institute. 2015;107:djv224.

[37] von Boehmer H, Daniel C. Therapeutic opportunities for manipulating T(Reg) cells in autoimmunity and cancer. Nature Reviews Drug Discovery. 2013;12:51–63.

[38] Blatner NR, Mulcahy MF, Dennis KL, Scholtens D, Bentrem DJ, Phillips JD, et al. Expression of RORgammat marks a pathogenic regulatory T cell subset in human colon cancer. Science Translational Medicine. 2012;4:164ra59.

[39] Gabrilovich DI, Ostrand-Rosenberg S, Bronte V. Coordinated regulation of myeloid cells by tumours. Nature Reviews Immunology. 2012;12:253–268.

[40] Tsoli M, Swarbrick MM, Robertson GR. Lipolytic and thermogenic depletion of adipose tissue in cancer cachexia. In Seminars in Cell & Developmental Biology. 2016;54:68–81.

[41] Nieman KM, Kenny HA, Penicka CV, Ladanyi A, Buell-Gutbrod R, Zillhardt MR, et al. Adipocytes promote ovarian cancer metastasis and provide energy for rapid tumor growth. Nature Medicine. 2011;17:1498–1503.

[42] Tang KD, Liu J, Jovanovic L, An J, Hill MM, Vela I, et al. Adipocytes promote prostate cancer stem cell self-renewal through amplification of the cholecystokinin autocrine loop. Oncotarget. 2015;7:4939–4948.

[43] Zhang Y, Daquinag AC, Amaya-Manzanares F, Sirin O, Tseng C, Kolonin MG. Stromal progenitor cells from endogenous adipose tissue contribute to pericytes and adipocytes that populate the tumor microenvironment. Cancer Research. 2012;72:5198–5208.

[44] Demir IE, Friess H, Ceyhan GO. Nerve-cancer interactions in the stromal biology of pancreatic cancer. Frontiers in Physiology. 2012;3:97.

[45] Magnon C, Hall SJ, Lin J, Xue X, Gerber L, Freedland SJ, et al. Autonomic nerve development contributes to prostate cancer progression. Science. 2013;341:1236361.

[46] Ferdousi M, Azmi S, Petropoulos IN, Fadavi H, Ponirakis G, Marshall A, et al. Corneal confocal microscopy detects small fibre neuropathy in patients with upper gastrointestinal cancer and nerve regeneration in chemotherapy induced peripheral neuropathy. PloS One. 2015;10:e0139394.

[47] Green ED, Watson JD, Collins FS. Human genome project: Twenty-five years of big biology. Nature. 2015;526:29–31.

[48] Liao XY, Lochhead P, Nishihara R, Morikawa T, Kuchiba A, Yamauchi M, et al. Aspirin use, tumor PIK3CA mutation, and colorectal-cancer survival. New England Journal of Medicine. 2012;367:1596–1606.

[49] Barcellos-Hoff MH, Lyden D, Wang TC. The evolution of the cancer niche during multistage carcinogenesis. Nature Reviews Cancer. 2013;13:511–518.

[50] Liu Y, Cao X. Organotropic metastasis: role of tumor exosomes. Cell Research. 2016;26;149–150.

[51] Peinado H, Aleckovic M, Lavotshkin S, Matei I, Costa-Silva B, Moreno-Bueno G, et al. Melanoma exosomes educate bone marrow progenitor cells toward a pro-metastatic phenotype through MET. Nature Medicine. 2012;18:883–891.

[52] Luga V, Zhang L, Viloria-Petit AM, Ogunjimi AA, Inanlou MR, Chiu E, et al. Exosomes mediate stromal mobilization of autocrine Wnt-PCP signaling in breast cancer cell migration. Cell. 2012;151:1542–1556.

[53] Maida Y, Takakura M, Nishiuchi T, Yoshimoto T, Kyo S. Exosomal transfer of functional small RNAs mediates cancer-stroma communication in human endometrium. Cancer Medicine. 2015;5:304–314.

[54] Sánchez CA, Andahur EI, Valenzuela R, Castellón EA, Fullá JA, Ramos CG, et al. Exosomes from bulk and stem cells from human prostate cancer have a differential

http://dx.doi.org/10.5772/66575

microRNA content that contributes cooperatively over local and pre-metastatic niche. Oncotarget. 2015;7:3993–4008.

[55] Ostman A. The tumor microenvironment controls drug sensitivity. Nature Medicine. 2012;18:1332–1334.

[56] Sun Y, Campisi J, Higano C, Beer TM, Porter P, Coleman I, et al. Treatment-induced damage to the tumor microenvironment promotes prostate cancer therapy resistance through WNT16B. Nature Medicine. 2012;18:1359–1368.

[57] Chen F, Qi X, Qian M, Dai Y, Sun Y. Tackling the tumor microenvironment: what challenge does it pose to anticancer therapies? Protein & Cell. 2014;5:816–826.

[58] Sun Y. Tumor microenvironment and cancer therapy resistance. Cancer Letters. 2016;380:205–215.

[59] Xu Q, Chiao P, Sun Y. Amphiregulin in cancer: new insights for translational medicine. Trends in Cancer. 2016;2:111–113.

[60] Sun Y, Nelson PS. Molecular pathways: involving microenvironment damage responses in cancer therapy resistance. Clinical Cancer Research: An Official Journal of the American Association for Cancer Research. 2012;18:4019–4025.

[61] Lotti F, Jarrar AM, Pai RK, Hitomi M, Lathia J, Mace A, et al. Chemotherapy activates cancer-associated fibroblasts to maintain colorectal cancer-initiating cells by IL-17A. The Journal of Experimental Medicine. 2013;210:2851–2872.

[62] Acharyya S, Oskarsson T, Vanharanta S, Malladi S, Kim J, Morris PG, et al. A CXCL1 paracrine network links cancer chemoresistance and metastasis. Cell. 2012;150:165–178.

[63] Nakasone ES, Askautrud HA, Kees T, Park JH, Plaks V, Ewald AJ, et al. Imaging tumor-stroma interactions during chemotherapy reveals contributions of the microenvironment to resistance. Cancer Cell. 2012;21:488–503.

[64] Roodhart JML, Daenen LGM, Stigter ECA, Prins HJ, Gerrits J, Houthuijzen JM, et al. Mesenchymal stem cells induce resistance to chemotherapy through the release of platinum-induced fatty acids. Cancer Cell. 2011;20:370–383.

[65] Duan CW, Shi J, Chen J, Wang B, Yu YH, Qin X, et al. Leukemia propagating cells rebuild an evolving niche in response to therapy. Cancer Cell. 2014;25:778–793.

[66] Johansson AC, Ansell A, Jerhammar F, Lindh MB, Grenman R, Munck-Wikland E, et al. Cancer-associated fibroblasts induce matrix metalloproteinase-mediated cetuximab resistance in head and neck squamous cell carcinoma cells. Molecular Cancer Research: MCR. 2012;10:1158–1168.

[67] Wang W, Li Q, Yamada T, Matsumoto K, Matsumoto I, Oda M, et al. Crosstalk to stromal fibroblasts induces resistance of lung cancer to epidermal growth factor receptor tyrosine kinase inhibitors. Clinical Cancer Research. 2009;15:6630–6638.

[68] Castoldi R, Ecker V, Wiehle L, Majety M, Busl-Schuller R, Asmussen M, et al. A novel bispecific EGFR/Met antibody blocks tumor-promoting phenotypic effects induced by resistance to EGFR inhibition and has potent antitumor activity. Oncogene. 2013;32:5593–5601.

[69] Saharinen P, Eklund L, Pulkki K, Bono P, Alitalo K. VEGF and angiopoietin signaling in tumor angiogenesis and metastasis. Trends in Molecular Medicine. 2011;17:347–362.

[70] Coppe JP, Patil CK, Rodier F, Sun Y, Munoz DP, Goldstein J, et al. Senescence-associated secretory phenotypes reveal cell-nonautonomous functions of oncogenic RAS and the p53 tumor suppressor. PLoS Biology. 2008;6:2853–2868.

[71] Courtwright A, Siamakpour-Reihani S, Arbiser JL, Banet N, Hilliard E, Fried L, et al. Secreted frizzle-related protein 2 stimulates angiogenesis via a calcineurin/NFAT signaling pathway. Cancer Research. 2009;69:4621–4628.

[72] Siamakpour-Reihani S, Caster J, Bandhu Nepal D, Courtwright A, Hilliard E, Usary J, et al. The role of calcineurin/NFAT in SFRP2 induced angiogenesis–a rationale for breast cancer treatment with the calcineurin inhibitor tacrolimus. PLoS One. 2011;6:e20412.

[73] Sun Y, Zhu D, Chen F, Qian M, Wei H, Chen W, et al. SFRP2 augments WNT16B signaling to promote therapeutic resistance in the damaged tumor microenvironment. Oncogene. 2016;35:4321–4334.

[74] Augustin HG, Koh GY, Thurston G, Alitalo K. Control of vascular morphogenesis and homeostasis through the angiopoietin-Tie system. Nature Reviews Molecular Cell Biology. 2009;10:165–177.

[75] Brunckhorst MK, Xu Y, Lu R, Yu Q. Angiopoietins promote ovarian cancer progression by establishing a procancer microenvironment. The American Journal of Pathology. 2014;184:2285–2296.

[76] Coppe JP, Boysen M, Sun CH, Wong BJ, Kang MK, Park NH, et al. A role for fibroblasts in mediating the effects of tobacco-induced epithelial cell growth and invasion. Molecular Cancer Research : MCR. 2008;6:1085–1098.

[77] McMillin DW, Negri JM, Mitsiades CS. The role of tumour-stromal interactions in modifying drug response: challenges and opportunities. Nature Reviews Drug Discovery. 2013;12:217–228.

[78] Straussman R, Morikawa T, Shee K, Barzily-Rokni M, Qian ZR, Du JY, et al. Tumour micro-environment elicits innate resistance to RAF inhibitors through HGF secretion. Nature. 2012;487:500–504.

[79] Wilson TR, Fridlyand J, Yan Y, Penuel E, Burton L, Chan E, et al. Widespread potential for growth-factor-driven resistance to anticancer kinase inhibitors. Nature. 2012;487:505–509.

[80] Jing H, Lee S. NF-kappaB in cellular senescence and cancer treatment. Molecules and Cells. 2014;37:189–195.

[81] Fuchs D, Metzig M, Bickeboller M, Brandel C, Roth W. The Gbeta5 protein regulates sensitivity to TRAIL-induced cell death in colon carcinoma. Oncogene. 2015;34:2753–2763.

[82] Liu F, Bardhan K, Yang D, Thangaraju M, Ganapathy V, Waller JL, et al. NF-kappaB directly regulates Fas transcription to modulate Fas-mediated apoptosis and tumor suppression. The Journal of Biological Chemistry. 2012;287:25530–25540.

[83] Sun Y. Translational horizons in the tumor microenvironment: harnessing breakthroughs and targeting cures. Medicinal Research Reviews. 2015;35:408–436.

[84] Teng MW, Ngiow SF, Ribas A, Smyth MJ. Classifying cancers based on T-cell infiltration and PD-L1. Cancer Research. 2015;75:2139–2145.

[85] Taube JM, Anders RA, Young GD, Xu H, Sharma R, McMiller TL, et al. Colocalization of inflammatory response with B7-h1 expression in human melanocytic lesions supports an adaptive resistance mechanism of immune escape. Science Translational Medicine. 2012;4:127ra37.

[86] Taube JM, Klein A, Brahmer JR, Xu H, Pan X, Kim JH, et al. Association of PD-1, PD-1 ligands, and other features of the tumor immune microenvironment with response to anti-PD-1 therapy. Clinical Cancer Research : An Official Journal of the American Association for Cancer Research. 2014;20:5064–5074.

[87] Gatalica Z, Snyder C, Maney T, Ghazalpour A, Holterman DA, Xiao N, et al. Programmed cell death 1 (PD-1) and its ligand (PD-L1) in common cancers and their correlation with molecular cancer type. Cancer Epidemiology, Biomarkers & Prevention : A Publication of the American Association for Cancer Research, Cosponsored by the American Society of Preventive Oncology. 2014;23:2965–2970.

Chapter 5

Patient-Centered Medicine and Self-Help Groups in Germany: Self-Help Friendliness as an Approach for Patient Involvement in Healthcare Institutions

Alf Trojan, Christopher Kofahl and Stefan Nickel

Additional information is available at the end of the chapter

http://dx.doi.org/10.5772/66163

Abstract

Collaboration between laypersons and professionals is closely linked to the concept of patient centeredness. Patient centeredness means meeting the needs of *individual* patients as well as reacting to patients' demands on the *collective* level. The support of self-help groups and their integration into healthcare institutions represent a major policy approach to fulfilling this requirement. Here, we first deal with the concept of patient centeredness in general, and the understanding of concept and use in Germany. We also provide a short definition of self-help friendliness (SHF) and discuss the success achieved in implementing it in Germany so far. We then clarify the closely related concepts of patient centeredness, patient participation and patient involvement SHF is seen as a strategy for increasing both patient centeredness and patient participation in healthcare services. We subsequently describe the involvement of self-help groups and patient associations in a series of empirical studies and practice-oriented projects carried out between 2004 and 2013. The last section contains a general discussion of the SHF approach as a means of systematically increasing sustainable patient centeredness and patient participation in healthcare services. Finally, we address the chances for future development in Germany and the transferability of SHF to other countries.

Keywords: self-help friendliness, self-help groups, patient centeredness, patient involvement, patient associations, healthcare institutions, healthcare research

1. Introduction

The backdrop to this chapter was the development and implementation of the concept of "self-help friendliness" (SHF) in Germany. This process started in 2004 and has good chances and prerequisites to be continued in the coming years. The idea behind is based on a number of expert opinions, surveys and well-documented model projects. Parallel to this practice-oriented developmental research, from 2008 to 2011, a research project with the title "Self-Help Friendliness as a Quality Concept" was carried out. The project was funded by the German Federal Ministry of Education and Research (BMBF) as part of a larger project in the BMBF's research framework program "Chronic Diseases and Patient Centeredness".

This chapter deals first with the role of SHF as one of the main elements in patient centeredness as well as its role in the overall German healthcare context. Thereafter, we concentrate on looking at the research and practical experiences gathered with the idea of SHF as well as outlining the present state of the concept's implementation in healthcare facilities.

2. Patient centeredness as a guiding concept

Providing a precise definition of and an approach to the concept of patient centeredness is challenging. Patient centeredness is no longer just a matter of treating patients in a "humane" manner; the concept has become very complex because of the fact that patients today are also evaluators, controllers, critics and active contributors to the development and regulation of the healthcare system.

This abandons any simple understanding of patient centeredness. However, until today the German Medical Association as one of the most important players in the German healthcare sector reduces patients' roles to more or less inactive recipients and beneficiaries. Their guideline on quality management in hospitals can be seen as an example how the term "patient centeredness" can be narrowed down to a number of unidirectional features of professionals towards patients, but not vice versa:

- "waiting times during admission to the hospital,
- receiving proper information during the doctor's visit,
- extent of care provided by nursing personnel,
- waiting times during X-rays, endoscopic examinations, laboratory exams, etc.
- handling of privacy concerns,
- wake-up and bedtime hours,
- contacts with social services,
- number and types of leisure programs,

- hygienic measures,
- guidance in the hospital, access to the parking lots and other means of assisting patients and visitors who enter the hospital" ([1] p. 45).

No doubt–all of these points are important. Nevertheless, the guideline gives the impression that the managers of health facilities knew in advance of how their organizations work and how their offers should be structured to ensure patient centeredness–and thus that they require no input on the part of the patients: "Patients trigger the demand for orientation, and the personnel takes the proper action" [2].

Even in differentiated and focused papers on patient centeredness in Germany, the contribution of the *active* patient in the concept of patient centeredness remains at least vague or is even completely absent (e.g., [3–5]).

A contemporary understanding of patient centeredness, however, demands just such active participation. Patient centeredness ought to balance the informational asymmetry between professional staff and patients and promote equitable interactions. It is not just a matter of sharing knowledge; also, the responsibility for therapy and diagnosis has to be distributed ensuring a reciprocal process to replace the former domination of the physician's perspective. This in turn demands great sovereignty and responsibility on the part of the patient [6]–not only on the microlevel of healthcare provision. It is a transforming perspective from the patient "who is cared for" to the patient who is an "active participant," and an active "creator of the treatment process" [7], and indeed of the entire provision of health and social services [8].

In 1995, the PubMed/Ovid MEDLINE system introduced the Medical Subject Heading (MeSH) term, "patient-centered care", defined as "design of patient care wherein institutional resources and personnel are organized around patients rather than around specialized departments" [9]. In 2001, the Institute of Medicine defined "patient centeredness" as: "health care that establishes a partnership among practitioners, patients and their families (...) to ensure that decisions respect patients' wants, needs and preferences and that patients have the education and support they require to make decisions and participate in their own care" ([10], p. 7). In his conclusion, Blum [11] summarized the concept of "patient-centered care" with the key-terms integration, information, communication and participation. Self-help-oriented patient centeredness corresponds to this modern definition by focusing on the cooperation of self-help organizations with professional services.

The International Alliance of Patients' Organizations (IAPO) did a systematic study to determine what patient centeredness looks like around the world [12]. Not surprisingly, they found many and manifold different definitions, which, however, have despite of their diversity very similar core statements. The definition supported by the IAPO is comparable to that of the Institute of Medicine [10]. In a declaration on patient-centered health care derived from that overview ([12], p. 29), the following five principles are given:

- respect
- choice and empowerment

- patient involvement in health policy
- access and support
- information

This understanding of patient centeredness is clearly reminiscent of the term "health literacy" propagated by the World Health Organization [13] as "the cognitive and social skills which determine the motivation and ability of individuals to gain access to, understand and use information in ways which promote and maintain good health". In this sense, patient centeredness is a continual companion in the endeavor to increase the health literacy of all citizens in general and patients in particular.

The concept of SHF runs parallel to the approaches put forward by the IAPO and the WHO. One of our original propositions is that the implementation of modern approaches to patient centeredness demands cooperation with self-help groups (see [14–16]). This thought is present in the newer secondary literature on patient centeredness, but does not play a prominent role in the light of the many other aspects of patient centeredness. Unfortunately, the various potentials for implementing self-help in patient centeredness have to date not been fully realized but often reduced to individual functions. Here, some German examples:

- classifying the complaints of self-help organizations as "patient feedback" ([177], pp. 62–63),
- regarding them as "complementary services" or as "complementary efforts" ([18], p. 25),
- relaying information on self-help groups during discharge procedures ([18], p. 19),
- "Using experiences of self-help" by allowing "persons concerned to assist in disseminating information to patients" ([17], p. 66),
- cooperation subsequent to hospitalization [18].

These forms of cooperation are oriented towards the short definition of patient centeredness as the "adjustment of available services and operating procedures to the presumed interests and needs of patients" [18].

More recently, the idea of participative (or shared) decision-making has played a major role. This thrust exists primarily in the individual doctor-patient relationship on the microlevel, from the patient vantage point as "co-production," and in the interactive process of decision-making [19]. In fact, however, there are a number of recent programmatic articles proposing a broader and more diverse understanding of cooperation. Some of the early demands and present opinions are reflected in the following research papers:

- Patients as "an important resource in the fight against ignorance, quality defects and waste in the healthcare system" [20].
- Quality is a utilitarian approach–meaning participation, i.e., "patients and insured persons are involved in decision-making processes at all levels through their position as users" ([21], p. 78).

- "We must give consumers of the healthcare system a voice and enable a dialog between them, the providers and the political system" ([22], p. 25).
- "Support for organized self-help is an area of activity that serves to strengthen citizen and patient centeredness" ([16], p. 24).
- The goal is to use the "collective competence" of self-help to influence new directions taken by caretaking structures and procedures, and generally to strengthen the skills of patients ([5], p. 1120).
- "Human relations should include and support all forms of self-help" ([17], p. 72).

The last quote refers to "patient-centered quality management" [17], which holds the promise of becoming a context for including cooperation with self-help groups in a less random way than offered by previous well-meaning but weak contacts.

The first important document that brought patient centeredness into the mainstream as a goal of continual quality management was an application developed in 1996 during the Conference of Health Ministers of the Federal States of Germany [23]; later found in the concordant application with the National Expert Council in Health Care [24]. At that meeting, "goals for a common quality strategy in the healthcare system" were adopted, the first goal being "systematic patient centeredness in the healthcare system".

The document clearly shows that concepts concerning patient centeredness and patient participation in the healthcare system are closely related with quality assurance strategies. To date, this has been realized to a greater extent for the macrolevel of the healthcare system [16] than for the mesolevel of individual institutions such as hospitals and physicians' offices ([25], p. 19).

Implementing a comprehensive plan for patient centeredness is greatly dependent on how sound the systems for quality management and quality assurance have been established. Groene et al. [26] did a Europe-wide study of hospitals concerning the relationship between patient centeredness and the presence of quality management: patient centeredness was more broadly implemented in hospitals with an extensive quality management.

Good quality management on its own, however, does not necessarily guarantee an implementation of patient centeredness–neither is it a predictor of systematic cooperation with self-help organizations. In addition to quality management, "proper overall conditions are necessary that allow those professionals working in the healthcare system to take patients into due consideration, in particular, by focusing on their wishes and preferences," as was formulated in the conclusion of the "Report on Citizen and Patient Centeredness in the Healthcare System" ([16], p. 26).

This short overview of the German situation serves to point up deficits and to provide suggestions on establishing cooperations with self-help groups. In our opinion, the concept of "self-help friendliness of healthcare services" comprises quite a number of advantages for patients and healthcare providers and should be integrated in a modern understanding of patient centeredness. During the course of implementation in Germany, some important milestones have been achieved:

- The basic principles of cooperation with organized self-help groups were systematically reduced to a manageable list of just seven quality criteria.
- Specific criteria were adapted to the individual areas of healthcare (inpatient, outpatient, public health, rehabilitation).
- The criteria for all areas were jointly formulated by healthcare professionals–predominantly those, who are responsible for quality management–representatives of self-help organizations, and professional staff of the self-help clearinghouses. The criteria represent the interests and needs of both the collective group of patients and their self-help representatives and professionals in the respective positions.
- Implementation was tested in all areas, systematic approaches were developed, and the concepts and experiences derived from these attempts were put at the disposal of all facilities involved (www.selbsthilfefreundlichkeit.de).
- The quality criteria comprise three main dimensions: (1) a coordinated cooperation based on information and support for the self-help groups; (2) the dimension of participation through information exchange, participation in the further education of staff, as well as participation in bodies such as quality circles and ethics committees; (3) the long-term assurance of communication and cooperation (sustainability). The completeness and applicability of these criteria were evaluated in a number of surveys and with various groups of participants [27, 28].
- The consistent application of these criteria leads to an overall increase in the systematic participation of organized self-help on the mesolevel. The participation of patients is generally accepted, but to date has not been realized in reforms of the healthcare system.
- Overall, this approach highlights previously neglected aspects of patient centeredness and cooperation with patient lobby groups. It demonstrates ways in which these aspects can be solidly integrated into quality management, both at the level of individual facilities and on the system level.

As the advantages of SHF discussed in this section are rather abstract so far, we will strive to present the relevant aspects in clearer and concreter terms. The next section systematically focuses on the relationship between the three main programmatic terms patient centeredness, SHF and patient participation.

3. On the relationship between patient centeredness, self-help friendliness and patient participation

Patient centeredness, SHF and patient participation are concepts with rather fuzzy borders. Presently, there are no agreed-upon scientific definitions. At least, the fact that these three terms represent the key concepts for creating healthcare that is tailored to patient needs and requirements, and thus likely also suited to ensure economic effectiveness, is globally accepted [29–38]. Internationally, there are a number of different approaches, methods and regulatory instruments for integrating patient participation into healthcare systems [39–43].

In Germany, the development and implementation of these concepts has gone hand in hand with the overall rise of the self-help movement and for some time has been subsumed under the catchword "Self-Help Friendliness". The only other similar country in this regard is Austria, which established a similarly important role for self-help within its healthcare system [44, 45]. Three factors in particular can explain the present development in Germany: First, there is a well-established landscape of self-help organizations and up to 100,000 self-help groups with around 3–3.5 million members. Second, this development has been supported systematically for several decades now [46], especially, by Para. 20 h of the Social Security Code, Book V, which requires that the statutory health-insurances companies pay EUR 1.05 per insured person to promote self-help, which sums up to around 73 million EUR. (This amount is changed every year to reflect cost-of-living increases). Third, since 2004, the German government has adopted a policy whereby patients (including for the most part the representatives of self-help organizations) are increasingly being included in the future planning of the healthcare system at the macrolevel.

Yet systematic cooperation between physicians and self-help groups as a way to increase patient participation as well as the quality of healthcare provided has barely been addressed in the international research literature. For this reason, we must rely on the ongoing discussion in Germany to determine the relations among the various different concepts.

It is helpful to differentiate between a broader and a narrow employment of the term patient centeredness. As mentioned at the outset, patient centeredness basically comprises everything that is carried out or improved upon within a healthcare facility to affect patient care. In accordance with the popular slogan "The Patient Is the Focus of Our Concerns," patient centeredness becomes nearly synonymous for comprehensive quality management.

The narrow understanding regards everything that directly concerns cooperation with patients and their welfare as belonging to patient centeredness. The broad understanding also includes the two components that make up this concept: "internal" and "external" patient centeredness [47]. *Internal* patient centeredness reflects all interventions that deal with the structures and processes occurring within a hospital which serve the well-being of the patient; *external* patient centeredness concerns everything that is in direct contact with patients and occurs in cooperation with the patient. This understanding of patient centeredness may also be seen as the invitation directed towards the patients to participate in the processes of professional caretaking.

The participation of the patients may be further divided up into different levels of intensity. Participation may reflect only "joint knowledge" (strengthening one aspect of health literacy), to "having a say" (participation in the relevant boards and committees) or up to "codetermination" (participation in the decision-making process and active voting rights in boards and committees).

All three basic concepts–patient centeredness, participation and SHF–are employed on all three levels: physician–patient interaction (microlevel), the institutional level of the individual facility (mesolevel) and on the system level of the entire healthcare system (macrolevel).

This chapter is concerned mainly with the mesolevel and the associated question: How can we create and anchor more SHF (and thus greater patient centeredness and participation) in the facilities of the healthcare system? We used an instrument from our research project to measure "self-help-related patient centeredness." This concept comprises two components: (1) strengthening *individual* self-help competences (How intensively does the hospital support individual patients by informing, enabling and including them in caretaking processes?); (2) strengthening *collective* self-help efforts (How intensively does the hospital cooperate with self-help groups in accordance with quality criteria?).

Within the context of this volume on patient-centered medicine, we barely touch on the microlevel and the macrolevel. Rather, our focus lies clearly on the *collective patient centeredness* on the mesolevel, that is, initiating cooperation between local health facilities and collective self-organized patient groups. SHF is considered one special aspect of the quality dimension "patient centeredness." SHF is only shortly discussed by us on the macrolevel, in particular when we are concerned with SHF in quality management systems (in this context: the so-called accreditation systems) and in the coordination of SHF at the national level ("Network Self-Help Friendliness and Patient Centeredness in the Healthcare System" [48]).

4. Developing the approach

The development of self-help friendliness did neither follow a "master-plan" nor a rigorously designed intervention concept. The process should rather be considered as a complex participative research program, which has been described in a recent publication more comprehensively [49]. The development comprised a number of empirical surveys and practice-oriented demonstration projects. All these projects were conducted between 2004 and 2013 (see **Table 1** [49]). Their methods differed considerably: most often qualitative (expert interviews and focus groups) and quantitative surveys were combined. As a guiding principle, patient representatives contributed in several stages of the research. Due to the participative approach, we proceeded only step by step. The core elements of self-help friendliness became continuously clearer by discussing the relevant quality criteria in the various sectors of health services. The implementation in one sector inspired and facilitated the process in the following ones. There was a steering group of professional self-help supporters, social scientists and staff from both sickness funds and healthcare providers, who looked for funding and decided on how to proceed. One milestone was the foundation of a network on SHF in 2009 (see Section 6.3). In its first years, the network consisted primarily of actors who had made major contributions to the support of self-help groups (SHGs) in various contexts and had promoted their recognition in practice and politics of healthcare provision. They favored a more systematic approach to sustainable collaboration between SHGs and healthcare professionals and were willing to find and/or to provide resources for implementing SHF. Particularly, healthcare insurance companies funded a number of both model projects and research. The steering group of healthcare insurance representatives and a professional self-help supporter have been the driving force for further development till today. They are

http://dx.doi.org/10.5772/66163

supported by a "federal coordination office" funded by a consortium of four sickness funds [48].

Study area (year)	Type of study	Sample	Main results
Hospital, part 1 (2004/2005)	Explorative survey	30 SHO, 20 SH clearing houses	Participative development of criteria
Hospital, part 2 (2004–2006)	Model project, implementation study	2 hospitals in Hamburg	Testing and final formulation of 8 criteria; 2 hospitals awarded "quality seal"
Hospital, part 3 (2008–2010)	Model project, implementation study	31 hospitals in NRW, 17 finishing the process	Process pattern and guidelines for becoming self-help friendly; 17 hospitals awarded distinction
Public health service (2009–2011)	Delphi method, interactive identification and approval of quality criteria	16 public health departments	10 quality criteria approved by workshop of public health doctors at their annual conference 2011
Ambulatory care (2009–2011)	Model project, implementation study	9 practices, individual MDs from 8 specialties	6 criteria approved and introduced into quality management manual for doctors in NRW
Rehabilitation (2010–2013)	Model project, implementation study prepared by focus group of 14 SHR	2 rehabilitation hospitals	5 criteria successfully tested; 2 hospitals awarded distinction; introduction in one national accreditation system planned

Abbreviations: SHO, self-help organization; SH, self-help; SHR, self-help representative.

Table 1. Major studies and steps in the development of SHF [49].

4.1. Development of self-help friendliness in hospital care

The concept of SHF stems from two sources. The first is a former survey of 345 contact persons out of 658 SHGs in Hamburg. As a main result of this research, it became clear that most SHGs were not satisfied with the care they have received. Consequently, they wanted changes both in the attitudes of their healthcare providers and in the running of healthcare institutions. These results were interpreted as a plea for intensified communication and collaboration between SHGs and professional staff in health services. Self-help friendliness was the most systematic approach to reach this goal.

The other source and stimulus for this approach were the annual "self-help forums", a sort of workshop of SHG members and medical doctors of all specialties. They are regularly organized by the Medical Chamber of Hamburg in collaboration with the local clearinghouse for SHGs. In the course of a discussion about shortcomings of hospital care, the idea of "self-help friendly hospitals" arose. It was appealing to both parties, doctors and self-help members. In 2003, this term resulted the first time in a formal cooperation statement between the Federation of Hamburg State Hospitals and SHGs. At the same time, the idea came up to initiate and to evaluate the implementation of the approach in some pilot hospitals. The funds for an explorative study and the process evaluation of the model project were granted in autumn 2004 from the Federal Association of Company Health Insurance Funds (BKK BV).

The explorative study started in 2005: A questionnaire was sent to self-help organizations and self-help clearinghouses with extensive experience in cooperation with healthcare providers, SHGs and SHOs, and patient representatives. About 30 organizations and 20 self-help clearinghouses administered the questionnaire. They responded to questions concerning their wishes and expectations and assessed several statements on quality criteria that had come up so far in the self-help forums. These assessments provided a first quantitative picture of what was important for self-help groups and, hence, what they would prefer to be implemented. This was the first basis for the identification and formulation of those quality criteria that were adopted in the end.

A steering group of the model project decided for the relevant criteria. The group comprised a project leader (a former self-help supporter with know-how in quality management), three hospital quality managers, two employees of the local clearinghouse and four members of SHGs. Staff members of the Hamburgian Institute of Medical Sociology accompanied the process as consultants. Eight criteria for good collaboration between hospitals and SHGs were developed [49]:

1. The hospital offers rooms, infrastructure and possibilities for public relations.
2. Patients of the hospital are personally informed about self-help on a regular basis.
3. The hospital supports public relations of the SHG.
4. The hospital appoints a staff member as a contact person for self-help.
5. Staff and SHG members meet regularly for information exchange.
6. SHGs are involved in further education/training of staff.
7. SHGs are involved in quality (control) circles and ethics committees.
8. The collaboration is formally agreed on and the activities will be documented.

Most of the criteria address the support of SHGs by the hospital; criteria 5–7 aim at a permanent and regular involvement of SHGs in the health service quality.

The implementation of self-help criteria was achieved in two hospitals in a process of nearly two years. Thus, the "reality-test" of the quality criteria was passed successfully. As a reward (and as an incentive for their further engagement), the two hospitals were awarded a "Quality Seal for Self-Help Friendliness" in 2006, based on an external audit. Eight members of SHGs, who had been trained for this task, played a major role in the on-site Visitation. The quality criteria were published in their final version as a brochure guiding and encouraging both hospital staff and self-help advocates in other places to do the same.

The process as a whole, however, had to face several delays due to lack of funding. Finally, the welfare organization "Der PARITÄTISCHE North Rhine-Westphalia" provided resources for the next development project from 2008 to 2010. This model project had the aim to develop a standard for the consecutive steps of implementing the quality criteria in hospitals, which resulted in nine steps of becoming "self-help friendly" [49]:

1. The agency for SHF (or a self-help clearinghouse) contacts and informs the hospitals.
2. First consultation of the agency takes place in the hospital.
3. The agency contracts the hospital and mediates contacts with self-help clearinghouses.
4. The staff of the self-help clearinghouses counsel hospital staff and mediates SHGs.
5. The hospital and SHGs collaborate in a quality circle.
6. Measures to fulfill the quality criteria are put into practice and are part of the internal quality management system.
7. The hospital applies for a certificate (optional).
8. The quality report of the hospital is signed by representatives of SHGs.
9. Certification (formally documented distinction) is awarded and can be used in public relations of the hospital.

Thirty-one hospitals in North RhineWestphalia (NRW) made use of the offered supportive consultations. Seventeen finished the implementation of SHF with a distinction in the form of a certificate. The capacities of the experienced facilitator for becoming self-help friendly (a half-time social worker), however, turned out to be overstrained: She did not have the resources and capacities to meet the total amount of requests for support, which means that probably more than the mentioned 17 hospitals might have finished the process if more resources were available.

The projects in Hamburg and in NRW produced decisive findings and downloadable guidance for other hospitals interested in becoming self-help friendly (www.selbsthilfefreundlich-keit.de). There were, however, some problems that obviously had to be conceived of as obstacles for further spreading the approach: For example, providing additional staff for consultations, as it was carried out in the model project during the implementation process, was too expensive. Consequently, the approach was changed in the sense, that near-by clearinghouses get a small amount of funding in order to compensate them for their additional workload. A formal quality seal after an external audit, which in the first project had seemed the most appropriate way to give an award, required too many resources, too, both human and (ultimately) financial: The expenditure of time was enormous, not only for the hospitals but also for the self-help representatives. Presently, healthcare services can gain an award of the network "Self-Help Friendliness and Patient Centeredness". Prerequisites are (i) a certification by patient representatives that at least one measure for each quality criterion was put into practice and (ii) the inclusion of the SHF quality criteria in the internal quality management system. These two simple requirements are easy to fulfill, and additionally guarantee that no advertising of SHF claims can be made without the consent of the collaborating SHGs.

4.2. Development of self-help friendliness in other areas of the health services

After successful implementation in the hospital area, the program was started in the other healthcare sectors: public health, practices and rehabilitation services.

The process in the area of public health did not correspondent to the general pattern because the ten quality criteria stem from an interactive process with professionals from 16 public health departments of local health authorities. Unfortunately, we do not have exact data on the degree of local self-help engagement.

The next project started to develop equivalent criteria for ambulatory care. The ten existing recommendations for cooperation and the eight quality criteria for inpatient care can be seen as the starting point for developing criteria for outpatient care in an interactive process of all relevant players. They produced a consensus document with six criteria that was accepted by the Association of Statutory Health Insurance Physicians Westphalia-Lippe. These criteria are quite similar in substance to those in the hospital sector.

Nine practices (doctors with their staff) participated in the process: general practice, gynecology and obstetrics, internal medicine, urology, ophthalmology, orthopedics, ENT medicine and pediatrics. At the end of the process, in which the medical and lay persons jointly developed measures to put the quality criteria into practice, the implementation of the criteria was formally documented in a report which was signed by both parties. The practices were subsequently awarded as being self-help friendly. Current endeavors are underway to build doctors' networks (instead of single practices) as partners in this process.

The way in hospitals for rehabilitation was similar to the hospital sector. It started with a team on quality assurance of an umbrella organization of rehabilitation institutions. In December 2011, the preliminary SHF criteria were discussed with 14 self-help representatives in a workshop. Result were five quality criteria which were tested in a pilot project with two rehabilitation hospitals. The participating SHGs in the project were: the Interest Group of Contergan Victims, the Federal Osteoporosis Association, the German Multiple Sclerosis Society and a local SHG of stroke patients. Finally, the successful implementation of SHF was proved by self-help representatives and led to a distinction for the hospitals involved.

5. Research limitations and transferability to other countries

It is not possible to discuss in detail the research limitations of all the mentioned pilot projects and studies. But, we would like to highlight some basic problems, both of which have been discussed in a previous medical sociological publication [50].

One of the most important features of the different studies is their participative and explorative nature. This has obviously some disadvantages: Despite all attempts to gather information as systematically as possible, and to reflect all aspects of the development, implementation, testing and evaluating of SHF, the results are not representative, neither for all healthcare professionals nor for all self-help representatives. Participants are usually highly motivated, therefore the results are emphasizing much more the positive factors rather than potentially negative ones. All generalization of these experiences and results is only adequate in comparable contexts with healthcare institutions which are open towards SHF and patient centeredness.

The very essential issue whether SHF is feasible *at all* in healthcare institutions can be answered positively. This implies that SHF criteria have been integrated into the quality management system of healthcare institutions and thus have become sustainable.

However, another question is the transferability to other countries. Though there are many other types of collaboration with patients [51], we only know about comparable approaches in Austria. This seems to be grounded in similarities both in the hospital sector and in the policies to promote and integrate self-help associations. Firstly, of course, due to the common language, which makes it much easier to adopt ideas and concepts, and secondly because of a regular exchange between Austrian and German members of relevant advisory boards. Regarding to the first German pilot project in Hamburg, similar initiatives of SHF have been put into practice in about 40 Austrian hospitals [44]. This confirms the transferability in comparable contexts.

6. Discussion and conclusion

6.1. Advantages of the concept

Cooperativeness is a necessary but not sufficient prerequisite for better involvement of civil society organizations into quality improvement of healthcare services. The SHF concept and its implementation offer some incentives, such as the formal acknowledgement, either as a "seal" for promotion and corporate identity or as a quality certificate in the framework of a quality management audit [52].

The additional practical support by counselors from the agency for SHF and the involved clearinghouses on self-help assist hospital staff and SHG members to find practical solutions for systematic implementation of collaboration. The open concept of patient centeredness and the "romantic vision" of a doctor-patient partnership turn into a measurable task. This intensifies the pressure to produce a positive result: Failing is visible and may be embarrassing.

Further advantages are several (positive) side effects which are coming up for both partners [50]:

- If a hospital decides for the SHF approach, this has to be communicated to patients. This leads to an overall reflection of questions like: 'What is self-help at all?', 'Is self-help beneficial or can it bear risks?', 'Can I recommend it to my patients and, if so, how shall I communicate it to them?'
- If SHGs decide for the approach, they will have to fulfill additional roles, and the "voluntary"-aspect of their work may become subordinated. Other questions arise: 'How do we define our (new) roles?', 'How do we make sure

that we are complementary to professional staff and are not regarded as a substitute?', 'How do we deal with dissatisfaction or conflicts between hospital patients and hospital staff?' etc.

In the whole, we can summarize that the discussion about and reflection of the topic "SHF" helps ...

- to inform healthcare professionals about the role, chances and possibilities of self-help and specifically their integration in professional care,
- to clarify the roles and responsibilities of healthcare staff and members of SHGs,
- to better understand the viewpoints and needs of their counterparts,
- to learn new facets of the relevant indication and their implications for coping, self-management and consequences in daily life.

These are all relevant aspects of (collective) patient centeredness which can measurably increase the quality of care in terms of health outcomes [53], better functional status, less infections, shorter hospital stay and higher compliance in joint replacements [54], or significantly reduced decubitus rates and other treatment-related complications [55]. Hospitals and quality managers like the effect that patient centeredness even can reduce the costs and thus increases the financial benefit [31].

There is some evidence that SHF is a solution to the lack of sustainable cooperation and a way to enhance quality standards in patient-centered care. There are signs that this results in better patients' health outcomes. Nevertheless, there is a strong plausibility that healthcare institutions will re-adapt their procedures to patients' needs and thereby improve patient satisfaction, self-management, coping and health literacy. Forster and Rojatz ([44], p. 50–51) scientifically accompanied the SHF-implementation process in Austria with a qualitative study design. They found some reasons why the approach is appreciated and accepted. Positive effects were mainly seen in the quality of cooperation with patients, better visibility and acknowledgement of SHGs, as well as an increasing patient centeredness in hospitals. Interestingly, the interviewed experts did not see any disadvantages. A qualitative study in Germany found strong agreement of both professional staff and SHG-members that SHF would enhance quality in care [56].

6.2. Shortcomings of the concept

We should not ignore that the voluntary engagement of SHG members can be rather limited due to their health conditions or even may stop suddenly because of decompensation or acute episodes of their illness [57]. Furthermore, healthcare organizations or legal committees require more and different skills beyond the "mere patient role". Just being a patient who is only describing his or her experience, but not reflecting the wider circumstances and the impact on healthcare providers, institutions, regulations and legislation, may not be sufficient for the concerted development of common strategies [58]. Finally, the motives of the different stakeholders addressing SHGs can be very different. SHGs seem increasingly to be a target of other actors in the health policy arena, like healthcare insurers or especially the pharmaceutical industry [59], but also scientists, predominantly in the area of medical research.

The study with 625 moderators of physicians' quality circles showed that doctors considered a possible relief of their workload as one of the strongest incentives [60]. However, there is a high probability that professionals like to establish patient groups as auxiliaries [61] rather than equal partners. Several scientists have expressed their concerns about such kinds of "misuse" and identity changes of patient groups; they argue professionals would offer collaboration but in fact try to get "control" of SHGs [62] or to achieve "colonization" [63–65].

Rabeharisoa's "partnership model" [61] should hinder misuse and legitimate SHGs to adjust any aberrations from SHF as it is meant by its proponents, if this concept is truly understood and adequately put into practice. However, also here, the above described risk remains: Professionals might take personal advantage of SHGs or could try to co-opt them.

6.3. Future development in Germany

The SHF approach is focusing at one global aim, which is to reach quality improvements in health care by promoting both individual and specifically collective patient centeredness. While at the *macro* level patient representatives and other stakeholders in the healthcare system mostly negotiate legal and administrative quality issues, SHF at the *meso*level deals significantly more with daily routines and practical issues in treatment and care. One crucial requirement can be seen in positive attitudes and mindsets of professional staff towards SHGs, which is not a matter of course, as still today some reservation against SHGs exists. Thus, SHF is also a continuous change management process.

The German Network "Self-help Friendliness and Patient Centeredness" promotes a nationwide cooperation between healthcare professionals and SHGs by developing and circulating training materials, implementing agencies for the support of SHGs, running pilot projects, and integrating self-help-friendly criteria into quality management and accreditation measures (www.selbsthilfefreundlichkeit.de). This network helps to tackle critical and non-desirable developments at an early stage, and it can deal with new ways and opportunities for dissemination. These are reaching from appropriate incentive structures to demonstration projects aiming at the implementation of patient centeredness and/or SHF in institutions [36, 39, 43].

The German network has grown steadily since its start in 2009. In April 2016, the network consisted of 118 active members, 42 of them were local self-help clearinghouses, 13 were sent by self-help organizations, 29 were coming from hospitals, and 16 from rehabilitation hospitals. Twenty-one general hospitals and 5 rehabilitation centers are currently distinguished as self-help friendly healthcare institutions. In each case, the list contains the names of the collaborating SHGs (about 9, on average; [66]). If we keep in mind that *active* dissemination is still in the beginning, these figures look promising.

6.4. Potential and barriers for international transfer and dissemination

Patient involvement and participation in health care and the ways and methods to integrate them in health policies vary in different countries. Despite comparable aims and principles in general, it is still difficult to compare these developments cross-nationally due to diverse and permanently transforming national healthcare systems [67]. At least for the Western World, we meanwhile can assert that there is a common agreement for the need of patient centeredness and patient involvement. We can also state that the reluctance and resistance of healthcare professionals against patients and SHGs, which has often been observed and discussed in the past [68], has more or less overcome. Nevertheless, it is still quite challenging to transfer models of good practice from one country to the other, not only because of the different healthcare systems themselves, but also because of different developments in health-related civil society organizations and in support systems for patients and/or SHGs.

The self-help support system in Germany is rather unique. No other country in the world provides such manifold professional support for patients and SHGs at regional levels. Three hundred clearinghouses and -offices for self-help are serving for around 100,000 SHGs, and several hundred further community-based information centers provide information and counseling for citizens and patients in consumer protection, care, legal affairs and patients' rights, etc. However, as research on self-help and patient involvement and the debates in these areas are usually held, written and published in German language, the German situation remains widely unknown in other countries except the German speaking like Austria or parts of Switzerland.

The characteristics of the German healthcare system with its integrated self-help support system have certainly promoted patient involvement and participation. The German Network "Self-help Friendliness and Patient Centeredness in the Healthcare System", initiated by stakeholders from all relevant healthcare areas, was an important and necessary measure for the development of systematic cooperation between healthcare providers and SHGs at the mesolevel [48].

The SHF-concept may possibly sound rather specific and seems strongly being influenced by the German legislations and circumstances. Nevertheless, there are some similarities with other approaches in other countries aiming at patient centeredness, at least concerning the individual (patient) level of patient centeredness rather than the collective (SHG) level. A study by Luxford et al. [35], for example, has recently investigated organizational barriers and facilitators towards patient-centered care in eight healthcare institutions in the USA. They conducted 40 qualitative interviews with healthcare professionals and stakeholders and shaped out nine key facilitators very similar to the quality criteria for SHF. Methods and measures may be different, but it seems obvious that change management towards patient participation, patient centeredness, public involvement or SHF needs participative approaches integrating patients and patient representatives–or specifically: self-help representatives–if a satisfactory cooperation between patients and professional healthcare staff is to be achieved. The German examples demonstrate that self-help and patient groups play an important role in further development of partnerships between patients and healthcare professionals and thus for improvements in the quality of healthcare services.

http://dx.doi.org/10.5772/66163

Author details

Alf Trojan, Christopher Kofahl and Stefan Nickel*

*Address all correspondence to: nickel@uke.de

Institute of Medical Sociology, University Medical Center Hamburg-Eppendorf, Hamburg, Germany

References

[1] Bundesärztekammer [German Medical Association], editor. Leitfaden: Qualitätsmanagement im deutschen Krankenhaus [Guidline: Qualiy Management in German Hospitals]. 3rd ed. München: Zuckschwerdt; 2001

[2] Bleses H. Patientenorientierung als Qualitätsmerkmal [online-dissertation]. Berlin: Humboldt-Universität. http://edoc.hu-berlin.de/dissertationen/bleses-helma-2005-01-24/html/index.html

[3] Stratmeyer P. Das Patientenorientierte Krankenhaus. Eine Einführung in das System Krankenhaus und die Perspektiven für die Kooperation zwischen Pflege und Medizin [The patient-centered hospital]. Weinheim, München: Juventa; 2002

[4] Hoefert HW, Härter M, editors. Patientenorientierung im Krankenhaus [Patient-centeredness in Hospital]. Göttingen: Hogrefe-Verlag; 2010

[5] Weis J et al. Patientenorientierung in der Onkologie. Konzepte und Perspektiven im Nationalen Krebsplan [Patient-centeredness in the Oncology]. Onkologe. 2011;17: 1115–1126

[6] Bauer U, Rosenbrock R, Schaeffer D. Stärkung der Nutzerposition im Gesundheitswesen - gesundheitspolitische Herausforderung und Notwendigkeit [Strenghtening the user position in the healthcare system]. In: Iseringhausen O, Badura B, editors. Wege aus der Krise der Versorgungsorganisation. Bern: Huber; 2005. pp. 187–201

[7] Sixma H. Quality of (Home) Care Services in the Netherlands. Past, Present, Future; 2006 [oral presentation]

[8] Engelhardt HD. Leitbild Menschenwürde. Wie Selbsthilfeinitiativen den Gesundheits - und Sozialbereich demokratisieren [Guiding Concept of Human Dignity]. Frankfurt / M: Campus; 2011

[9] http://www.ncbi.nlm.nih.gov/mesh?term=patient-centered%20care [Accessed: 2016-07-12]

[10] Hurtado MP, Swift EK, Corrigan JM, editors. Envisioning the National Health Care Quality Report. Committee on the National Quality Report on Health Care Delivery,

Board on Health Care Services: Institute of Medicine. Washington: National Academy Press; 2001

[11] Blum K. Patientenzentrierte Versorgung – ein Blick ins Ausland. [Patient-Centered Care–A View of Abroad]. Slide Presentation, Berlin; 7.4.2011

[12] International Alliance of Patients' Organizations (IAPO), editor. What is Patient-Centred Healthcare? A Review of Definitions and Principles London: IAPO; 2006

[13] Commission on Social Determinants of Health (CSDH), editor. Achieving Health Equity: From Root Causes to Fair Outcomes. Geneva: WHO; 2007

[14] Stark W. Selbsthilfe und PatientInnenorientierung im Gesundheitswesen – Abschied von der Spaltung zwischen Professionellen und Selbsthilfe? [Self-help and Patient-centeredness in Healthcare] In: Borgetto B, Troschke J, editors. Entwicklungsperspektiven der gesundheitsbezogenen Selbsthilfe im Deutschen Gesundheitswesen. Deutsche Koordinierungsstelle für Gesundheitswissenschaften. Freiburg; 2001. pp. 47–66

[15] Robert-Koch-Institut (RKI), editor. Selbsthilfe im Gesundheitsbereich. Gesundheitsberichterstattung des Bundes, Themenheft 23 [Self-help in Healthcare]. Berlin: RKI; 2004

[16] Robert-Koch-Institut (RKI), editor. Bürger - und Patientenorientierung im Gesundheitswesen. Gesundheitsberichterstattung des Bundes, Themenheft 32 [Public and Patient Involvement in Healthcare]. Berlin: RKI; 2006

[17] Sänger S. Patientenorientiertes Qualitätsmanagement [Patient-centered Quality Management]. In: Hoefert HW, Härter M, editors. Patientenorientierung im Krankenhaus. Göttingen: Hogrefe Verlag; 2010

[18] Hoefert HW, Härter M. Einleitung: Patientenorientierung [Introduction: Patient-Centeredness]. In: Hoefert HW, Härter M, editors. Patientenorientierung im Krankenhaus. Göttingen: Hogrefe Verlag; 2010

[19] http://www.patient-als-partner.de/index.php/english/start.html [Accessed: 2015-19-03]

[20] Dierks ML, Schwartz FW. Einleitung [Introduction]. In: Dierks ML, Bitzer EM, Lerch M, Martin S, Röseler S, Schienkiewitz A, Siebeneick S, Schwartz FW, editors. Patientensouveränität. Der autonome Patient im Mittelpunkt. Working Paper; 2001

[21] Hart D. Bürgerbeteiligung: Zum Konzept und seinen rechtlichen Rahmenbedingungen [Public involvement: concept and its legal frameworks]. In: Badura B, Schnellschmidt H, editors. Bürgerbeteiligung im Gesundheitswesen – eine länderübergreifende Herausforderung – Ideen, Ansätze und internationale Erfahrungen. Forschung und Praxis der Gesundheitsförderung, Bd. 10, 2nd ed. Köln; 2001. p. 73-80

[22] Badura B. Beteiligung von Bürgern und Patienten im Gesundheitswesen [Participation of citizens and patients in healthcare]. Bundesgesundheitsblatt – Gesundheitsforschung – Gesundheitsschutz. 2002;45:21–25

[23] Gesundheitsminister-Konferenz (GMK). Ziele für eine einheitliche Qualitätsstrategie im Gesundheitswesen [Goals for a common quality strategy in the healthcare system]. Beschluss der 72. GMK am 9./ 10.06.1999 in Trier

[24] Sachverständigenrat für die Konzertierte Aktion im Gesundheitswesen, editor. Gutachten [Expertise] 2000/2001: Bedarfsgerechtigkeit und Wirtschaftlichkeit. Bd. I: Zielbildung, Prävention, Nutzerorientierung und Partizipation; Bd. II: Qualitätsentwicklung in Medizin und Pflege; Bd. III: Über-, Unter - und Fehlversorgung. Baden-Baden: Nomos (Bundestagsdrucksache 14/5660, -5661, -6871); 2012

[25] Gerlinger T. Nutzerorientierung im Gesundheitswesen – Probleme und Perspektiven [User Involvement in Healthcare – Problems and Prospects]. In Mozygemba K et al., editors. Nutzerorientierung - ein Fremdwort in der Gesundheitssicherung? Bern: Huber; 2009. pp. 17–29

[26] Groene O et al. Is patient-centredness in European hospitals related to existing quality improvement strategies? Analysis of a cross-sectional survey (MARQuIS study). Quality & Safety in Health Care. 2009;18(Suppl I):i44–i50

[27] Trojan A, Nickel S. Integration von Selbsthilfefreundlichkeit in das Gesundheitswesen – Entwicklungen und Perspektiven [Integration of self-help associations into the health services system–developments and perspectives]. Das Gesundheitswesen. 2011;73(2): 67–72

[28] Bobzien M, Trojan A. Selbsthilfefreundlichkeit" als Element patientenorientierter Rehabilitation – Ergebnisse eines Modellversuchs [Self-help friendliness as an element of patient-centered rehabilitation–Results of a pilot project]. Rehabilitation. 2015;54:1–7. doi:10.1055/s-0034-1398515

[29] Akrich M, Nunes J, Paterson F, Reharisoa V. The Dynamics of Patient Organizations in Europe. Paris: Collection Sciences Sociales; 2008

[30] Allsop J, Jones K, Baggott R. Health consumer groups in the UK: a new social movement? Sociology of Health and Illness. 2004;26(6):737–756

[31] Charmel PA, Frampton SB. Building the business care for patient-centered care. Healthcare Financial Management. 2008;62(3):80–85

[32] Conklin A, Morris ZS, Nolte E. Involving the Public in Healthcare Policy. An Update of the Research Evidence and Proposed Evaluation Framework. Santa Monica: RAND Corporation; 2010

[33] Engelhardt HD, Trojan A, Nickel S. Leistungen von Selbsthilfegruppen und deren ökonomische Bewertung [Performance of self-help groups and their economic evaluation]. Bundesgesundheitsblatt: Selbsthilfe. 2009;52:64–70

[34] Lewin S et al. Interventions for providers to promote a patient-centred approach in clinical consultations. Cochrane Database of Systematic Reviews. 2001;(4):CD003267 doi:10.1002/14651858.CD003267

[35] Luxford K, Safran DG, Delbanco T. Promoting patient-centred care: a qualitative study of facilitators and barriers in healthcare organizations with a reputation for improving the patient experience. International Journal for Quality in Health Care. 2011;23(5): 510–515

[36] Shaller D. Patient-Centered Care: What Does It Take? New York: The Commonwealth Fund; 2007

[37] Taylor K. Paternalism, Participation and Partnership–The Evolution of Patient-centeredness in the Consultation. Patient Education and Counselling. 2009;74(2): 150–155

[38] Epstein RM, Fiscella K, Lesser CS, Stange KC. Why the nation needs a policy push on patient-centered health care. Health Affairs. 2010;29(8):1489–1495

[39] Bitton A, Martin C, Landon BE. A nationwide survey of patient-centered medical home demonstration projects. Journal of General Internal Medicine. 2010;25(6):584–592

[40] Box G. Patient participation groups: the national picture. Quality in Primary Care. 2009;17(4):291–297

[41] Canadian Health Services Research Foundation. CHSRF Patient Engagement Project–PEP. http://cahspr.ca/en/funding-opportunity/chsrf-patient-engagement-project-%E2%80%93-pep [Accessed: 5th March 2011]

[42] Bovenkamp HM van de, Trappenburg MJ, Grit KJ. Patient participation in collective healthcare decision making: the Dutch model. Health Expectations. 2010;13(1):73–85

[43] Scrivens E. Widening the scope of accreditation–issues and challenges in community and primary care. International Journal for Quality in Health Care. 1998;10(3):191–197

[44] Forster R, Rojatz D. Selbsthilfegruppen als Partner der Gesundheitsförderung im Krankenhaus. Eine Analyse am Beispiel krankenhausbezogener Kooperationsprojekte [Self-help Groups as Partners für Health Promotion in Hospitals]. Institut für Soziologie, Universität Wien. Forschungsbericht; 2011

[45] Forster R, Braunegger-Kallinger G, Krajic K. Selbsthilfeorganisationen als "Stimme der Patienten": Erfahrungen und Herausforderungen von Interessenvertretung und Beteiligung [Self-help Organizations as "Voice of Patients"]. In: Meggeneder O, editor. Selbsthilfe im Wandel der Zeit. Frankfurt/Main: Mabuse; 2011. pp. 9–39

[46] Geene R, Huber E, Hundertmark-Mayser J, Möller-Bock B, Thiel W. Entwicklung, Situation, und Perspektiven der Selbsthilfe-Unterstützung in Deutschland [Development, Situation and Perspective of Self-help Support in Germany]. Bundesgesundheitsblatt – Gesundheitsforschung – Gesundheitsschutz. 2009;52:11–20

[47] Körner M, Ehrhardt H, Steger AK. Interne und externe Patientenorientierung in der medizinischen Rehabilitation [Internal and External Patient-centeredness in the Medical Rehabilitation]. Public Health Forum. 2011;19(70):21–22

[48] http://www.selbsthilfefreundlichkeit.de [Accessed: 2016-07-06]

[49] Nickel S, Kofahl C, Trojan A. Involving self-help groups in health care institutions: the patients' contribution to and their view of "self-help friendliness" as an approach to implement quality criteria of sustainable cooperation. Health Expectations. 2016. doi: 10.1111/hex.12455 (March 2016)

[50] Kofahl C, Trojan A, Knesebeck Ovd, Nickel S. Self-help friendliness: a German approach for strengthening the cooperation between self-help groups and health care professionals. Social Science and Medicine. 2014;123:217–225

[51] Keizer B, Bless R. Pilot Study on the Position of Health Consumer and Patients' Organisations in Seven EU Countries. Den Hague: ZonMw; 2010

[52] Trojan A, Werner S, Bobzien M, Nickel S. Integration von Selbsthilfezusamenschlüssen in das Qualitätsmanagement im amulanten und stationären Versorgungsbereich [Integration of self-help associations into the quality management of outpatient and inpatient health care]. Bundesgesundheitsblatt: Gesundheitsforschung – Gesundheitsschutz. 2009;52:47–54

[53] Meterko M, Wright S, Lin H, Lowy E, Cleary PD. Mortality among patients with acute myocardial infarction: the influences of patient-centered care and evidence-based medicine. Health Services Research. 2010;45(5):1188–1204

[54] Di Gioia AM. The AHRQ Innovation Exchange: Patient - and Family-centered Care Initiative Is Associated with High Patient Satisfaction and Positive Outcomes for Total Joint Replacement Patients. Rockville: Agency for Health Care Research and Quality; 2008

[55] Isaac T, Zaslavsky AM, Cleary PD, Landon BE. The relationship between patients' perception of care and measures of hospital quality and safety. Health Services Research. 2010;45(4):1024–1040

[56] Schumann M. Die Institutionelle Verankerung von Selbsthilfe im Krankenhaus. Fördernde und hemmende Rahmenbedingungen aus Sicht der beteiligten Akteure [The Institutional Entrenchment of Self-Help in Hospitals. Facilitating Factors and Barriers from the Stakeholders' View]. MH Hannover: Magisterarbeit Public Health; 2011

[57] Matzat J. Selp-help/mutual aid in Germany–a 30 year perspective of a participant observer. International Journal of Self-Help and Self Care. 2006–2007;5:279–294

[58] Berger B, Gerlach A, Groth S, Sladek U, Ebner K, Mühlhauser I, Steckelberg A. Competence training in evidence-based medicine for patients, patient counsellors, consumer representatives and health care professionals in Austria: a feasibility study.

Zeitschrift für Evidenz, Fortbildung und Qualität im Gesundheitswesen. 2013;107(1): 44–52

[59] NAKOS, editor. Transparenz und Unabhängigkeit der Selbsthilfe [Transparency and Independence of Self-help]. Wahrung der Selbstbestimmung und Vermeidung von Interessenkonflikten. Berlin: NAKOS Konzepte und Praxis 6; 2012

[60] Nickel S, Trojan A, Kofahl C. Increasing patient centredness in outpatient care through closer collaboration with patient groups? An exploratory study on the views of health care professionals working in quality management for office-based physicians in Germany. Health Policy. 2012;107(2):249–257.

[61] Rabeharisoa V. The struggle against neuromuscular diseases in France and the emergence of the partnership model of patient organisation. Social Science & Medicine. 2003;57:2127–2136

[62] Borkman T. Groups at the turning point: emerging egalitarian alliances with the formal health care system? American Journal Community Psychology. 1990;18(2):321–32

[63] Kelleher D. Self-help groups and their relationship to medicine. In: Kelleher D, Gabe J, Williams J, editors. Challenging Medicine. London: Routledge; 2006. pp. 104–121

[64] O'Donovan O. Corporate colonization of health activism? Irish healthadvocacy organizations' modes of engagement with pharmaceutical corporations. International Journal of Health Services. 2007;37(4):711–733

[65] Marent B, Forster R, Nowak P. Conceptualizing lay participation in professional health care organizations. Administration and Society. 2015;47(7):827-850. doi: 10.1177/0095399713489829

[66] http://www.selbsthilfefreundlichkeit.de/selbsthilfe/content/wie_wir_auszeichnen/ausgezeichnete_kliniken/index_ger.html [Accessed: 2016-07-06]

[67] Burau V. Transforming health policy and services: challenges for comparative research. Current Sociology. 2012;60(4):569–578

[68] Moeller ML. History, concept and position of self-help groups in Germany. Group Analysis. 1999;32(2):181–194

Chapter 6

Holistic Care Philosophy for Patient-Centered Approaches and Spirituality

Nilufer Demirsoy

Additional information is available at the end of the chapter

http://dx.doi.org/10.5772/66165

Abstract

Holistic care philosophy, acknowledging the existence of a very close relationship between body, mind and soul (spirit) and focusing on individualism, emphasize that every dimension of human is distinctive and unique as well as they are also connected to each other. While integrity value is defined as an important concept for personal development and health; providing treatment and healing by holistic approach extends to Hippocrates, the founder of medicine. It is emphasized in this philosophy that holistic approach is important for individuals and as well as physical ailments, spiritual effects of illness need to be investigated. Spirituality, one of the components of the holistic approach, takes "belonging to the community" into account. Spirituality is concerned with "growth," and it is the essence of existence and congenital according to this approach. It is an instinctive (genetous) awareness for helping someone else. Individual's perception of his own spirituality increases his inner peace and personal satisfaction. Health-care professionals should have environment and proximity, capable of offering holistic medical care services, for understanding patient's sociocultural and psychological situation as well as being closely acquainted with patient's family and life environment. Because this concept is individualistic, and an aspect of human arising from his multidimensional experiences. Undoubtedly, during these applications, it is also important to show the respect for autonomy of thought and belief basically in the context of principle of "not harming." If it is acted responsibly in fulfillment of this approach, a good level of medical discipline, spirituality and science integration will be reached. The studies to be performed in this field will offer new opportunities for understanding the great mysteries of life and medicine better and for development of medical care services.

Keywords: holistic care, spirituality, patient-centered approach

1. Introduction

Patient-centered approach, the level of increasing competition, technology, education, logistics and communication opportunities of our age made it necessary to focus on the expectations and desires of the patients in health care. With the humanistic approaches in the health care, the necessity has increased even more. And with the patient-centered approach, it became the contemporary approach, which is regarded as the presentation of the health care.

The patient-centered approach is an approach, which guarantees the patient values in clinical decisions at a certain extent and is respectful of the individual preferences, needs and values of the patient. The approach does not only guarantee the patient in informing them of diagnosis, treatment and healthy behaviors. Also, it does not mean that the patients must be provided with whatever they desire. What is expected in patient-centered approach is the guidance from health professionals. The patient should be provided with information about the alternatives, benefits and risks thoroughly and unbiased accompanied by guidance. This signifies that the patient's cultural tendencies and traditions, individual preferences and values, family conditions, social environment and lifestyle are taken into account. The fundamental basis of the patient-centered approach is the holistic approach. When the etymological origin of the holistic approach is analyzed, it can be seen that the word derives from "holism."

Holism, eng: holism, fr: holisme, ger: holismus. Holism is the common term for the philosophical approaches emphasizing that the whole is greater than the sum of its parts. According to the approach, the whole cannot be understood by analyzing its component parts. The components that help us to see and to hear the reality constitute the whole. When viewed from this aspect, the holistic approach also applies to the field of medicine. While the concept of holism was first defined in the 1890's; in 1926, in the medical field, J. Smut in his work titled "Holism and Evolution" stated that "the world has been managed by a holistic process, in which the forms of substance increase continuously and new wholes are being formed" [1] and explained by noting that medical holism has individualistic, societal and environmental aspects. Human is considered to be part of the universe, nature, and supernature, in which they exist. In this perception, the spirit and body are designed with disease and health. The value of integrity is a significant concept for self-improvement and health. Therapy and cure with the holistic approach date back to 5000 years ago. Hippocrates (460 BCE-370 BCE), known as the founder of the medical science, emphasized that the holistic approach is significant and the spiritual effects of the disease must be considered. He emphasized this by saying "It is more important to know what sort of person has a disease than to know what sort of disease a person has" [2].

Hippocrates said, "The natural healing power inside us is the most important source for recovery." The duty of the doctor is to stimulate the healing power before giving a therapeutic substance [3]. As Galileo said: "You cannot teach a man anything, you can only help him find it within himself."

A holistic approach is regarded in a variety of different respects of the holistic care. However, what is fundamental in the holistic approach is that the health professionals should be able to evaluate and view the patient as an entire "individual," not just as an individual with a disease. Humans are valuable; above all, they are just humans. The human is an entity with the most developed intelligence among the living beings and who can think, reason, communicate and plan for the future. So, the human is honorable. Human is an entity different in many other respects (intelligence, apprehension, memory, imagination, expression, opinions, speech, morals, modesty, curiosity, anxiety, happiness, regret) and has superior qualities and skills thanks to these respects in general. People, possessing integrity, are born, grow, age and die after living on earth for some time. People should be evaluated and treated with holistic approach due to their nature when required. In order for a quality service to be provided in the field of health, a health professional is expected to be a good listener, a good speaker, a fine thinker, understanding and feeling of the emotions of the others with good recommendations. When the modern medicine, developing technology, insufficiency of the health-care systems, rise in the diseases, changes in the climatic conditions, the fact that the health-care professionals work intensively and under stress are taken into account, it has become a complex system, in which the physicians are unable to spare sufficient time for the patients [4, 5].

In the philosophy of holistic care, focusing on the individualism, which acknowledges that there is a strong relationship between body, mind and spirit, it is emphasized that every aspect of the human dimension is uniquely single as well as interconnected with each other. While the integrity, value is defined to be a significant concept for the self-improvement and health, it emphasizes that the spiritual effects of the illnesses along with the physical disorders must also be examined. In the philosophy of holistic care, the holistic treatment and care approaches along with the holistic diagnosis must be evaluated together.

In the concept of holism within the philosophy of holistic care, the physical and spiritual needs should be prioritized without ignoring the medical treatment applications. It can be stated that meeting the psychosocial needs effectively among these needs has a positive contribution in decreasing the physical needs and as well as increasing the effectiveness of the medical treatment. According to the World Health Organization, the health is a state of complete physical, mental and social well-being. Health is the harmony between the body, mind and spirit. Therefore, the holistic health of the individual is possible with the implementation of all the treatment types including spirituality [6].

Spirituality is an effort to understand and acknowledge the individual's relationships between themselves and other humans, their function in life and the meaning of life. At the same time, it is the result of knowledge gained throughout life and involves elements meaningful to an individual, which makes the purpose of life [6–8]. A variety of different definitions are used regarding spirituality (**Table 1**). When providing nursing services, knowing these concepts will be guiding for professionals [9].

Spirituality is one of the elements of holistic approach takes the principle "belonging to the society" into account. In this approach, "growth" relates to spirituality and the essence of existence and is inherited.

A sacred journey (Mische 1982)
Individual's life principle or basis (Clark et al. 1991)
Explanation of the radical truths (Legere 1984) and ultimate values (Cowley 1997)
Meaning and purpose of life (Legere 1984, Clark et al. 1991, Fitchett 1995, Sherwood 2000)
Being bound with unconditional love (Ellison 1983, Clark et al. 1991, Ross 1997)
Loyalty to him/herself (Reed 1992) and loyalty to others (Sherwood 2000)
Relationship between the mystery, great power, God, universe or life (Reed 1992)
Beliefs of the individual regarding the world (Soeken and Carson 1987)

Table 1. Definitions of spirituality

It is an (inherited) innate awareness to help others. Individual's comprehension of their own spirituality, increases internal peace and individual's own pleasure. Spirituality is the learning and changing process as a result of supreme power and individual relationship. A person first understands and apprehends his/her own inner ego, then with the help of this knowledge, decides and implements their expectations and desires. A person, who can successfully execute this as it is supposed to be, that is, a person, who can comprehend their ego, may understand their environment, the incidents and people better [8, 10]. When evaluated from this perspective, it can be seen that the majority of the holistic medicine applications tend to promote this belief and ego. According to another definition, "Spirituality is the learning and changing process as a result of an individual relationship." In the twelfth century, spirituality was defined so as to determine the psychological aspect of the human life in contrast to its physical aspect, to demonstrate the religious human in the fifteenth and sixteenth centuries, in the seventeenth century with its contemporary meaning for the first time in France, and in the twentieth century with its religious and nonreligious meanings. Nowadays, it is considered to be a broad concept rather than being bound to a traditional religion for many people. Since the spiritual dimension has a strong effect on factors relating to health, attitudes and behaviors, it is accepted to be the "fundamental element" of the philosophy of holistic care [10, 11].

If spirituality is defined in contextual conditions, spirituality means a human's search for a relationship with a spirit and it is his/her expression of this. Spiritualism expresses a metaphysical notion, according to which the universe is based on a spiritual basis, and the substance is independent of the spirit. Spiritualism can be defined as "unifying power" affected by the body and spirit and affects the body and spirit at the same time.

Spiritual care/approach is the inclusion of the beliefs, which are helpful in coping with the physical and spiritual difficulties and particularly the emotional needs of the individual; self-education and self-actualization approaches to the treatment process. While in the World Medical Association Declaration of Lisbon (1981) [12], it is stated that "The patient has the right to receive or to decline spiritual and moral comfort, including the help of a minister of his/her chosen religion"; in the World Medical Association Declaration of Amsterdam (1994) [13], it is stated that "Everyone has the right to have his or her moral and cultural values and religious and philosophical convictions respected." Moreover, in the same declaration the statement

http://dx.doi.org/10.5772/66165

"Patients have the right to enjoy support from family, relatives and friends during the course of care and treatment and to receive spiritual support and guidance at all times" and in the European Charter of Patients' Rights Basis Document (2002) [14] the statement "Article 12- Right to Personalized Treatment: Each individual has the right to diagnostic or therapeutic programs tailored as much as possible to his or her personal needs" emphasizes the spiritual care right.

It is important that the nurses take the concept of spirituality into account within the nursing plans, for which they are responsible for performing when delivering health care [15].

Spirituality is confused with many concepts. When the similarities and differences between concepts are specified, it will be possible to explain spirituality better. When spirituality and similar concepts are explained:

The lexical meaning of the word belief is being bound to an idea, believing in a religion, belief in a thing, notion or discipline. In addition to these, it also means a fixed notion since it has been accepted widely and an established general opinion [6, 8, 16–18]. James W. Fowler defines the word belief as a component of the main motivations of the individuals oriented towards life in its most general sense. When evaluating the belief development process, Fowler does not only emphasize the relational nature but also the imaginary nature. Fowler states that there is a significant relationship between the comprehension and evaluation forms of the human, and surrendering to the belief and imagination methods. Fowler believes that the belief is universal, unique to the human being's nature and correlated with human's interpretation process [19].

Spirituality is the sum of everything that the individual is associated with beyond the material and the intrinsic sources regarding their central meanings. Spirituality can also be defined as making an effort for the meaning of life, its purpose and the inner peace without any God belief beyond a religious dependence. Spirituality is also defined as a high level of belief, becoming divine or the infinite power of energy [11, 20]. Not all the concepts of spirituality are associated with a religion. In an evaluation relating to spirituality, it is seen that the majority of the modern conceptions are in line with one of the three categories. (1) God-centered spirituality, regarded as the motivation for the notion and practice in theologies and envisioned to be wide or narrow; (2) earth-centered spirituality emphasizing the correlation between an individual and ecology or nature and (3) humanistic (human-centered) spirituality emphasizing the success or potential of the human. Thereby, spirituality is seen to be a multidimensional structure [21].

The dimensions of the spirituality is a matter, which focuses on making an effort to be in harmony with the universe, striving to find the answers about infinity, and individual's focus on emotional distress, physical disease or death [11, 20].

Religion derived from the Latin stem religio, meaning the relationship between the human and a greater power than human. The researchers specified at least three historical definitions of this term: (1) supernatural power, in which individuals are motivated or tied, (2) an emotion emerging in an individual who apprehends such power and (3) the ritualistic behaviors that are done for this power. In the study conducted by Wilfred Cantwell Smith (1962–1991), it is put forth that the religion has been gradually materialized, in other words, religion, which is mostly an abstract process, is turned into a concrete matter through a certain system (for example, religious groups, theological traditions, major world religions, etc.). According to Heschel, religious thinking "is an intellectual effort beyond the depths of reasoning. Religious thinking is a mental source for grasping the inside story of the final problems regarding the human existence [21]. It is a societal institution, which systematizes believing in God, supernatural powers, diverse divine beings; a piety, and an organization, which provides and consolidates in the form of beliefs, rules, institutions, ethics and symbols. Religion is also defined as a system, which anticipates a lifestyle for believers and involves the sacred and metaphysical values or the concept of God within the belief system.

2. What is the level of religiosity in Turkey?

In a survey conducted with 21,600 participants across 12 regions of Turkey, while 99.2% have been found to define themselves as Muslim, 4‰ as non-Muslim. 5‰ did not answer the question. 98.7% have been found to have no suspicion of the existence of God. About 96.5% of the participants agreed with the statement that the verses of Quran are true and valid in all times 96.5% agreed with the statement that humans will be resurrected and questioned after death, whereas 1% disagreed. About 42.5% of the participants across Turkey state that they pray five times a day; while 16.9 never pray. About 83.4% across Turkey express that they fast if they are in a good state of health. 2.5% never fast. 7.3% do not fast due to health status. While 11.7% of the participants melt lead and pour it into cold water to not be touched by an evil eye, 79.3% do not believe that it is beneficial. It was found that 64.9% shape their lives according to the rules of the religion. About 50.7% of the participants indicate that the most significant criteria of religiosity are to have faith in god, worship in complete and lead a life in line with the Islamic ethics. About 37% report that believing in God and being pure in heart is enough for religiosity, whereas 7.9% define religiosity as worshipping and praying on sacred days [22].

3. What is the level of religiosity in the United States?

Even though the religious beliefs and rituals are commonly practiced in the United States, it is seen that their implementation and evaluation are less common in the medical applications. In a Gallup Poll conducted in 2008 in the United States, it was found that 78% stated that they believed in God and 15% in a higher spirit. In a study conducted in 2010, it was found that 77% of the Americans identified themselves as Christian, 5% with a non-Christian tradition, 43% reportedly attended religious services at least once a week and 18% did not have an explicit religious identity.

4. What is the level of religiosity in the Europe?

In a survey conducted across the country in 2013, 26% of the respondents claim that religion is important in their own lives and 22% claim it is fairly important [23]. According to a Gallup poll conducted in 2011, 53.48% of the British claim that they are Christian and 7.22% said that they belonged to other faiths, whereas 39% said they had no religion. In 2015, the poll was repeated and 49% of the participants said they were Christian, whereas 42% said they had no religion. In 2011, a poll was conducted in Scotland and 56% of the respondents said they were not religious and only 35% said they were religious. According to the 2014 survey conducted in nine European countries, a majority of the population believes that did not think that a belief in God was a necessary part of being moral. This figure was as high as 85% in France and 80% in Spain [24].

5. Spiritual approach and spiritual care

Spirituality can be considered as the first component of the religion; however, it is a very broad term, which cannot be limited only to religious beliefs and applications. Spiritual beliefs or values may or may not be correlated with an organized religion. Besides, people without strong religious beliefs have spiritual dimensions as well. Spiritual values and beliefs are concepts beyond a belief in the power and consist of beliefs subjects such as health, death, sin, life after death and responsibility for others. It is a traditional, ritual and specific doctrine different than that of religion spirituality. Spiritualism is a lot more comprehensive than the religious applications, however, may include religious applications as well [7, 8, 20].

Spiritual needs are needs that promote the spiritual power of an individual or reduce the spiritual deprivation. Humans can meet these needs by means of relations with humans or God. Spiritual needs can be defined as trust, hope, love, truth, need for finding out the meaning and purpose of life, relationships, forgivingness, creativity, experiencing, need for emotional feelings (tranquility, comfortableness), need for speaking, consolation, rituals, praying and worshipping [6, 20].

Spiritual needs and applications are very important concepts for many patients; however, they are ambiguous terms for the health professionals. Throughout history, the doctors have been trained to diagnose and treat disease and received little or no education regarding the spiritual dimension of the patient. In addition to this, it has been alleged that the professional ethical approach permits the doctor to implement their professional practice but not to question the patient's beliefs, and the deficiency in the concept is tried to be explained as such. When the deficiency is combined with the differences in societal beliefs, religious rituals and spiritual applications, a wide range of belief systems emerge. As a matter of fact, no doctor is expected to comprehend the individual applications of different belief systems. What is expected is necessary sensitivity since individual needs may show variations.

When conditions that may arise as a result of spirituality is addressed, it is understood that while the spiritual values help individuals feel themselves better, the spiritual distress occurs in a group of individuals, who are having trouble with their belief and value system, which gives meaning to life and brings hope and power, or in a group of individuals who are at risk. Spiritual distress occurs when the individual's values and beliefs are under threat in the environment they live in or the individual is in an existential crisis. Spiritual distress emerges at times when the individual is in a despair condition or unable to find a reason to live. The individual feels a moral gap. Besides, as a result of spirituality, conditions such as spiritual pain, spiritual alienation, spiritual anxiety, spiritual guilt, spiritual anger, spiritual loss, spiritual despair, disappointment, displeasure, gap, regret, guiltiness, grief may emerge [25].

Health is the harmony between body, intelligence and spirit. Therefore, in order to help the individual to protect and sustain the integrity of their existence, a care system (medical and nursing care), which will ensure the care of individual's existence, should be implemented. The fundamental care functions are to protect and enhance health, prevent diseases and relief pain. Thanks to this point of view, providing care for the spiritual dimension of an individual must be part of the fundamental functions of the health professionals. Individual's needs such as hope, finding the meaning and purpose of life, love and belonging to somewhere are their spiritual needs and in this case, it is a therapeutic application for health professionals to listen to the individual's concerns, empathize with the individual and respond these needs. It is important to evaluate all the humans with this perspective and plan approaches, which will enhance the health of the individual holistically.

There are many effective factors for the spiritual approach to be included within the care services. The opinion system, spiritual needs and comprehending the physical care, hope for health, willingness and sensitivity, which are particularly at the center of the care service among the factors, has been effective. However, the conducted studies show that the patient's spirituality has been ignored and the spiritual care is insufficient (Wong and Lee 2008; [27]). The researchers state that the most important reason for the lack of spiritual care is the time constraint and educational deficiencies. According to a study conducted on nurses, the nurses both consider the issue about spirituality and spiritual care important and meet the work requirements (only 15.5% of the nurses and midwives have obtained information on spiritual care and 33.3% claimed that they have never heard the term spiritual care) [26, 27].

There are significant principles, which must be taken into account, regarding spiritual care.

These are as follows:

1. It must be aimed to explain the power of individual regarding the spiritual needs as much as the existing and potential problems.

2. The primary purpose of the health professionals in spiritual care must be to evoke the spiritual sources of an individual.

3. Spiritual care must be planned to respond to the spiritual needs of an individual, not to alter their beliefs or change their perspective.

4. Spiritual diagnosis and care must be built upon a reliable and sensitive relationship between the patient and physician. The care must be planned so that it would involve the culture, social and spiritual sources of the individual as well as their idea and religious applications.

5. When sharing information about the patients among team members, they must be aware of the personal limitations.

6. The importance of mentioning the spiritual care in health applications in written must be taken into consideration and the necessary regulations must be established [11].

The studies suggest that the religious beliefs and spiritual applications of the patients are important factors when deciding to cope with diseases and even in termination of life and in the resolution of ethical dilemmas regarding treatment options. It has been found that determining the spiritual beliefs of the patients during the healing process (with correct questions and independent of our own belief systems within the communication process) is very helpful and easier when giving explanatory information regarding the treatment process and its results [23, 28]. Research shows that religion and spirituality are associated positively with better health and psychological well-being [28–30]. Recent research also shows that patients involved in "religious struggle" have a higher risk of mortality [31]. Thus, physicians need to inquire about the patient's spirituality and to learn how religious and spiritual factors may help the patient cope with the current illness, and conversely when religious struggle indicates the need for referral to the chaplain.

The idea that there is a correlation between the tendency towards spiritual needs and religiosity is a popular belief around the world. However, it can be stated that this is not directly correlated with delivering the health care and religiosity.

6. It is important to include spirituality into the health applications

Religion and spiritual beliefs play an important role for many patients. When illness threatens the health, and possibly the life of an individual, that person is likely to come to the physician with both physical symptoms and spiritual issues in mind. Humans grapple with common issues of infirmity, suffering, loneliness, despair and death while searching for hope, meaning and personal value in the crisis of illness [32].

Religion is generally understood as a set of beliefs, rituals and practices, usually embodied within an institution or an organization. Spirituality, on the other hand, is commonly thought of as a search for what is sacred in life, one's deepest values, along with a relationship with God, or a higher power, that transcends the self. Persons may hold powerful spiritual beliefs and may or may not be active in any institutional religion. Spirituality can be defined as "a belief system, focusing on intangible elements that impart vitality and meaning to life's events."

Many physicians and nurses have intuitive and anecdotal impressions that the beliefs and religious practices of patients have a profound effect upon their existential experiences with illness and the threat of dying. Recent research supports this notion.

It has been found that when patients face a terminal illness, religious and spiritual factors often figure into their coping strategies and influence important decisions such as the employment of advance directives, the living will and the Durable Power of Attorney for Health Care [23, 33, 34]. In such cases, it is very important to determine the necessary comforting factors for the patient to trust the higher power and cope with the existing crisis.

In another survey, whereas 77% of patients like to have their spiritual issues discussed as a part of their medical care, <20% of physicians currently discuss such issues with patients. Around 50 medical schools now offer "spirituality and medical approach" elective course. The evidence in the medical literature that suggests a strong relationship between spirituality and medicine is increasing [35]. In a conducted study, it was found that religion and spirituality had positive effects on physical health and the nurses had a tendency to believe spirituality as a religious need.

According to a study conducted with 1800 patients by Dr. Herbert Benson from Mind/Body Medical Institute, the conclusion that there is a direct correlation between prayer and healing the illnesses. According to the studies conducted in the United States and the UK, it was discovered that praying reduces the symptoms and accelerate the healing process. According to the study conducted by Michigan University, the depression and stress are less likely to be experienced by religious people, whereas according to the study conducted by Rush University of Chicago, the premature death rate is found to be 25% less when compared with those who are not affiliated with a religion. In another study conducted on 750 patients, who had angiography, by Duke University, "the healing power of prayer" was scientifically proven. It was revealed that the cardiac patients that pray have 30% less mortality rate few years after the surgery. The chaplains prayed for 466 cardiac patients, receiving treatment at St. Luke's Hospital, and as a result the patients who were prayed for healed 11% faster and their disease symptoms reduced. According to the study conducted by Columbia University, people with reproductive problems were regularly prayed for. The fertilization success rate in these people rose to 16% from 8%. The growth rate of the healthy embryo rose to 50% from 25%. In another study conducted on 393 cardiac patients by the Hospital of San Francisco, 150 patients were regularly prayed for and it was revealed that the patients, prayed for by strangers, responded to the pharmacotherapy faster [36, 37].

It has been shown in many studies that the spiritual dimension has a clear effect on health, wellness and quality of life [27, 38, 39]. In the study conducted by Strang et al. [40] in Sweden, it was found that 98% of the nurses considered the spiritual care as necessary and 48% provided spiritual care. In the study made by Narayanasamy (2001), it was discovered that the nurses were not enough aware of the spiritual needs of the patients and emphasized that there was a lack of background information on creating the nursing care scheme about the spiritual care [40].

According to the survey conducted to determine the spiritual values by Wong et al. [27], it was found that the spirituality sub-dimension level was high; however, it was also noted that spirituality should not only be affiliated/evaluated with a religion.

In some studies, the effects of the spiritual well-being, hope and mood are focused upon. Fehring et al. (1997) defined the correlation between spiritual well-being, religiosity, hope and depression and determined the positive mood of the elderly individuals, whose religiosity and spiritual well-being is at a high level, were at a high level. Post-White et al. (1996) discovered that the spiritual and religious hope were influential in 32 cancer patients, who defined hope on the whole [40]. It has been revealed in a study that more than 40% of the 248 cancer patients stated that they got rid of their fears, found the meaning of life, refreshed their hopes and felt vigorous when their seven spiritual needs were met [15]. The researchers carefully examined spirituality and chronic diseases and determined that spirituality was a strong source in order to overcome problems regarding health. It has been discovered in a study on 35 hemodialysis patients that hope, worship and trust in God have an important role in defense mechanism. In a study conducted on patients with arthritis, it was found that they stated that belief in God is an important factor in their well-being. In another study, worship and faith were found to be a very significant source for the cancer patient [9]. In a study conducted on colorectal cancer patients, it was shown that high level of spiritual well-being is effective in the treatment of the major physical symptoms. It has been stated that patients' experiences with cancer increase their spiritual awareness, which is part of themselves [15, 41].

Spirituality has a critical importance in patient-centered care when coping with the disease during the diagnosis and the treatment period, survival, relapse and death processes of the cancer patients. Spiritual needs, spiritual distress and spiritual well-being affect the quality of life [42, 43]. The spiritual needs of patients with advanced cancer are found to be 72%, and it was stated that the spiritual needs are not supported enough in health care [43]. Being with family was the most frequently cited need (80.2%), and 50% cited prayer as frequently or always a need. Around 26% of the patients cited at least one unmet spiritual need [44]. Hsiao et al. stated that the four most cited spiritual needs during the semi-structured interview by the patients was, hope to survive and have a tranquil state of mind (88%), make life livable and protect dignity (88%), experience mutual human affection (100%), get help for a peaceful death (85%) [45]. In the compilation, in which the psycho-spiritual well-beings of the advanced cancer patients and patients who faced a terminal illness was examined by Lin and Bauer-Wu, they have specified particularly six main themes: self-awareness, effective coping with stress, engagement with others, sense of belief, sense of trust and the meaning of life/hope [46].

On the other hand, there are studies that emphasize adopting religious rituals and approaches or thinking intensively about religion may have negative effects on some patients and results [31]. There could be times that the disease will result in death or approach the terminal period, struggling with religion may play an important role. Patients who feel alienated from God, unloved by God, or punished by God, or attribute their illness to the work of the devil were associated with a 19–28% increased risk of dying. A study of religious coping in patients undergoing allogeneic stem cell transplants also suggests that religious struggle may contribute to adverse changes in health outcomes for transplant patients. In such cases, professional support will positively affect the clinical results [31, 47]. In this regard, it is emphasized that the spiritual care units founded in a health unit, provided significant results for the patients since they worked in cooperation with the doctor [48].

It has been emphasized in a study conducted on nurses and midwives that it is significant for the nurses, who have knowledge of spirituality and spiritual care concepts, to provide their patients with spiritual care for the knowledge to be implemented. It was found in the study that the concepts of spirituality and spiritual care are new concepts in the field of nursing, the nurses and midwives did not receive sufficient information regarding spirituality and spiritual care during their training and did not provide spiritual care. It was revealed that the nurses and midwives were affected by receiving information and providing the patient with spiritual care as a result of their scores on the spirituality and spiritual care evaluation scale. Therefore, it is recommended to include spirituality and spiritual care concepts within the nursing and midwifery training curriculums and regulate on-the-job training programs, intended for developing the awareness, knowledge, and applications of the nurses and midwives on holistic care's spiritual dimension [6].

In another study conducted in Turkey, it was found that the nurses lacked knowledge regarding the concept of spirituality and had a tendency to consider the spirituality as part of religious needs. Thus, the importance of providing enough knowledge to the members of the health-care team on spiritual and religious needs of the patients was emphasized during their training [49]. In the study conducted by Yılmaz and Okyay [50], it was discovered that 34.8% of the nurses obtained information regarding spirituality and spiritual care. While 70.3% defined the concept of spirituality correctly, 93.4% defined the concept of spiritual care correctly. In the study, 33.3% of the nurses and midwives claimed that they have never heard the concept of spiritual care [50].

In the study conducted by Çelik et al. [51], it was found that the nurses' comprehension of spiritual care affects the spiritual care service as well. There are new studies concerning spiritual care other than the field of nursing in Turkey. First of all, "1st National Psychology of Religion and Spiritual Care Workshop" was organized. "Cooperation Protocol Intended for Providing Spiritual Support in Hospitals" signed between the Presidency of Religious Affairs and the Ministry of Health on 01/07/2015. During the signing of the protocol, it was stated that the Ministry of Health has been cooperating with the Presidency of Religious Affairs since 2012, and case studies from Europe and the United States have been examined. After the chaplains are trained with the required knowledge, the spiritual support service will be provided to the patients and patient's relatives for the first time through the pilot scheme in some cities [52].

7. What should be done when determining the spiritual needs of the patients?

It has been emphasized in many studies around the world that there is a necessity for identifying the needs for spiritual care and evaluating spiritual/moral distress. Even though there are many scales in the literature regarding the matter, they need to have a conformability and validation between cultures when identifying the spiritual needs.

HOPE questions, which were developed to help to initiate the spiritual evaluation process during the meeting/medical anamnesis for doctors, are significant in qualitative aspect for the statements to be evaluated. They are confirmed by a survey by the researchers who developed it. This specific approach enables the general spiritual sources and concerns of the individual to be expressed with open-ended statements [35].

HOPE Questions are officially used for spiritual evaluation by doctors. First clue: H is related to the basic fundamental spiritual sources of the patient without directly focusing on spirituality or religion. Sources of hope, meaning, comfort, strength, peace, love and connection. This approach enables the patient to communicate on a variety of significant matters. Here, spirituality involves significant contacts, which are excluded from the limits of traditional religion, or covers people who have somehow drifted apart the religion. It allows some to express the concepts of prayer or god explicitly and voluntarily. There are many ways to ask questions in this regard and identify it. The second and third letters are O and P. It shows the area of assessment made to determine the importance of religion in patients' lives and the most beneficial applications for individual spirituality. If the answer to this question is "Yes," the inquisition should continue with questions concerning religion and individual spirituality. If the answer to this question is "No" and the patient seems to be comfortable, the physician either could conclude the inquisition or try to elaborate on the matter by asking "Isn't it important for you at all?" If the answer to this question is "Yes;" the physician may ask so now "What has changed?" in order to discuss the spiritual anxieties, which may have an impact on the medical care of the patients. The last reminding letter is "E." The matters concerning the medical care and termination of life are about the spiritual effects and beliefs of the patient. These questions might be especially helpful in the clinical care service level to an extent that they could be used in clinical management. They could also be beneficial for the patients, who are in the oncological treatment process, or patients with chronic diseases [35].

In the approach recommended to be used in the care processes of the nurses:

Listening to the patients statements concerning their spiritual tendencies;

1. Patient's statements about god, higher power, prayer, religious places (church, mosque, etc.) and religious leaders.

2. Evaluation of the observable signs on the patient and their room regarding the spiritual tendencies; spiritual books (Bible, Quran, etc.) and symbols (cross, etc.).

3. Evaluation of the anxiety (concern) symptoms; discouragement, worry, weakness/insufficiency in participation the daily spiritual applications, patient's statements regarding their concerns about god or higher power.

4. Evaluation of the spiritual distress symptoms: A communication process must be sustained taking into account the statements as follows: crying, sign of guiltiness, sleep disturbances, lack of spiritual trust, feeling of alienation from god or higher power, anger against health professionals/family/god or higher power, refusal of the belief and value systems, losing the meaning and purpose in life [15].

Individuals with spiritual perspective must be respected in health care; the health professionals must protect the fundamental principle autonomy and ensure the benefit-damage balance when determining the treatment and care plan, prepared for the patients. The implementation of the treatment and care scheme must be paid attention as part of the individual's respect principle. All the medical rehabilitative services delivered to the individuals must be implemented within the fundamental ethical principles. Even though the individual's respect principle is based on a secular foundation, it cannot be isolated both from the perception of the value of the health professionals and the patients, especially from the disease conditions.

There is always a person, who needs the value system, identified as the god or higher power. Accepting this as a fact or not ignoring it means the completion of the patient's physical, emotional, social and spiritual care. Thus the value judgments, which the patient has for their spiritual well-being, are their integral part. The protection of the existence of this integral part is the most fundamental way to respect.

8. Hospitals should work with the spiritual care specialists

The doctor needs a teamwork formed by well-educated chaplains/spiritual care specialists, who are trained to help the patient in a hospital. It is encouraging for a doctor to let their patients know that they are not alone concerning their spiritual needs; however, doctors may also be unauthorized in terms of spiritual needs. The majority of the chaplains in hospitals in the United States are now board certified and qualified personnel, who received training for communication. Rev. Director of Chaplaincy at Seattle Cancer Care Alliance describes the requirements for chaplains as follows:

1. Board Certification Objective Requirements
2. Seventy-two semester hours/108 quarter hours Masters in theological studies
3. One full-time year equivalent in clinical pastoral education (CPE) (ACPE residency)
4. Ordained or commissioned by a religious/spiritual tradition (accountability) (e.g., Christian, Jewish, Muslim, Hindu, Buddhist, Sufi, Sikh, Interfaith)
5. Endorsed by a religious/spiritual tradition for chaplaincy (accountability) [23].

Humans are indisputable beings due to their existence. The value of human beings does not decrease when they are diseased or it is hard to be granted for them or cannot be ignored. The high-speed change and differentiating needs have been more on the front lines when eliminating the illnesses. The coping methods should be included in the spiritual needs as part of the holistic health applications. Spiritual needs are considered to be an unavoidable part of the global health system as an evaluation scope. Both the doctors and patients have some difficulties in understanding the concept of spiritualism from this aspect within the societal organization. The studies and discussion, which will be made regarding this matter, will be a significant step for creating awareness. Since the beginning of history, the existence of spirituality within the holistic approach is as important as the other components since its sensitivity to the diseased individual and the support it provides during the healing process. It was scientifically proven that alienation from the patient-centered approach in medical applications for a certain period of time had negative effects on the patients. It has been intensively discussed again to include the holistic approach and its components in the medical applications.

In the recent history, there was a legal gap on delivering the spiritual services oriented towards either inmate or outpatient. In 2016, the cooperation protocol was formed, which was intended for delivering "spiritual care and religious consultancy services in hospitals." Within the limits of this protocol, six pilot cities including Ankara were identified and spiritual care units were formed and chaplains began to provide service. In the spiritual care unit, the patients and patients' relatives are provided with spiritual values such as patience, meditation, prayer/ implementation of some rituals related to beliefs and spiritual approaches with religious themes like destiny/sense and belief of existence. The implementation is a significant step for our country. It is insufficient and unilateral. It is necessary to scientifically emphasize the importance of this approach, in which the medical services are included, can be carried out by the health professionals, who has a qualification to talk with the patients and their relatives, and it even must be performed [52].

In this aspect, implementing the spiritual care applications effectively and efficiently, receiving wide acceptance and correct planning of the studies plays a crucial role. First of all, it is necessary that the health professionals, who are going to deliver this service, must believe the significance of this concept and form the correct approach methods for the patients. Therefore, primarily it is necessary for the health professionals to; (a) Possess the psychological counseling skills, (b) Possess the fundamental health knowledge, (c) Grasp the illness psychology, (d) Use the effective communication skills and (e) Be dominant over the religious literature, grasp the religious and cultural values of the community they live in. When delivering the health care, a sincere approach, and environment, which can deliver the holistic medical care services oriented towards understanding the sociocultural and psychological state of the patient along with understanding the family of the patient and the environment they live in, must be developed. In the course of these applications, it is very important to maintain the respect for the autonomy of thought and belief as part of the fundamental principle "no-harm." Whether the health professionals are a member of a religion or not, their beliefs and value judgments may affect the physician-patient relationship. In this bilateral condition, the physician should never ignore the individual respect principle for the patient. The fundamental purpose of the health professionals is to listen and talk to the patient.

The health professionals are as free as the patients on practicing their own belief and value judgments. The majority of the times the problem is not being able to put limits on the patients when determining the patients' needs and discussing their condition and patients' responses with instructions or obstructions. The health professionals refraining from these, mostly prefer to ignore patients' these needs.

If this approach is executed with responsibility, it will be a significant improvement in the medical discipline, spirituality and science integration. The studies, which will be conducted, will offer new opportunities to both develop the medical care services and to understand the great mystery behind life and medicals.

9. Obstructions which emerge when discussing the spiritual matters

Some doctors may find some reasons to prevent the controversies on the spiritual beliefs, needs and benefits of the patients. The reasons why the doctors do not discuss these matters are an improper environment, lack of knowledge on spiritual issues, or the variety of religious statements due to different cultures. Since the doctors do not possess any training on how to manage the meetings with their patients regarding this matter remains as one of the biggest obstacles. Occasionally, the doctors may have to approach the patients tolerably in order not to violate the ethical and professional limits or impose their own ideas on the patients.

In 2004, *JAMA*'s curricular survey showed that: "in 1994, only 17 of the 126 accredited US medical schools offered courses on spirituality in medicine. By 1998, this number had increased to 39, and by 2004, to 84 schools" [53].

In 1998, Association of American Medical Colleges (AAMC) developed medical school objectives related to spirituality and cultural issues. Regarding this matter, the prospective physicians are expected to improve themselves with the help of spiritual and cultural program.

Beyond the 4 years of medical school, residency programs, particularly, those with a primary care focus and a palliative care focus, are incorporating education in spirituality training residents. In addition, Continuing Medical Education (CME) events are now offered to practicing physicians through a series of annual conferences on "Spirituality in Medicine," the first of which was hosted by Harvard Medical School with Herbert Benson, MD, as a facilitator. Since 2008, Dr. Puchalski has directed an annual Spirituality and Health Care Summer Institute sponsored by the George Washington Institute for Spirituality and Health (GWISH) in Washington D.C. [23].

10. Conclusion

The patient benefits from a physician, they trust in and get support from. In the medical applications from past to present, the necessity of three fundamental combinations has been emphasized, the modern, classical medicine, biomedical medicine, holistic consciousness-based medicine. Holistic medicine, focusing on the spirit and self-ego, reveals the sense of life and the world and particularly the hidden and secret sources and power inside the patient. All three approaches form a combined whole. The holistic approach is unavoidable and necessary, particularly in diseases whose process is long and painful. In studies conducted in this aspect, it is seen that some approaches, implemented taking into account the spiritual past of the person, can be carefully examined. There are some issues, which must absolutely be discussed: Are patients' beliefs are important? Do they have a set of rituals related to their beliefs? Do these require limitations? The spiritual emotions patients are feeling must be evaluated. In this respect, when supporting the patient, aid must absolutely be received from the spiritual care specialists and sometimes from the chaplains. How the spiritual problems of the patient should be taken into consideration must be evaluated with the patient. There are some issues which need to be clarified: How can the spiritual care applications be influential/efficient and receive general consent? How to correctly plan the studies in this aspect? Who can primarily provide this service and what kind of training they need to have? The spiritual care studies should be conducted interdisciplinary and under a single roof. Psychology, Psychological Counseling and Guidance, Psychiatry, Social Services, Psychology of Religion and Health Sciences must be a strong liaison with each other.

Author details

Nilufer Demirsoy

Address all correspondence to: npoyraz@ogu.edu.tr; nilufer_p2@hotmail.com

Department of History of Medicine and Medical Ethics, Faculty of Medicine, Eskisehir Osmangazi University, Eskisehir, Turkey

References

[1] Demirsoy N, Değirmen N, Kırımlıoğlu N. The place and ımportance of the concept of holism in health services: review (in Turkish). Turkiye Klinikleri J Med Ethics. 2011;19(3):164–74.

[2] Freeman JT. A definition of holism. Br J Gen Pract. 2005;55(511):154–5.

[3] Owen MJ, Holmes CA. Holisim in the discourse of nursing. J Adv Nursing. 1993;18(11): 1688–95. doi:10.1046/j.1365-2648.1993.18111688.x

[4] Demirsoy N. Holistic medical practices reflected from ancient civilizations to our day: review (in Turkish). Turkiye Klinikleri J Med Ethics 2014;22(3).

[5] http://www.bravewell.org/content/Downlaods/What_Is_IM_2011.pdf [Accessed: 2016.08.07].

[6] Kostak MA. Spiritual dimension of nursing care (in Turkish). Fırat Sağlık Hizmetleri Dergisi. 2007;2(6):105–15.

[7] Çetinkaya B, Altundağ S, Azak A. Spiritual care and nursing (in Turkish). Adnan Menderes Üniversitesi Tıp Fakültesi Dergisi. 2007;8(1):47–50.

[8] Sulmasy DP. Spiritual issues in the care of dying patients: "…it's okay between me and god". JAMA 2006;296(11):1385–92. doi:10.1001/jama.296.11.1385

[9] Narayanasamy A. Spiritual coping mechanisms in chronically ill patients. Br J Nursing 2002;11:22, 1461. doi:10.12968/bjon.2002.11.22.10957

[10] Wigglesworth C. SQ-one skills of spiritual intelligence (in Turkish). Trans: Seda Toksoy. İstanbul: Kural Dısı Yayınları. 2013. p. 63–125.

[11] Ergül S, Bayık A. Nursing and spiritual care (in Turkish). C.Ü.Hemsirelik Yüksek Okulu Dergisi. 2004; 8(1):37–45.

[12] http://www.wma.net/en/30publications/10policies/l4/ [Accessed: 2016.06.04].

[13] http://www.who.int/genomics/public/eu_declaration1994.pdf [Accessed: 2016.05.07].

[14] http://ec.europa.eu/health/ph_overview/co_operation/mobility/docs/health_services_co108_en.pdf [Accessed: 2016.08.03].

[15] Taylor EJ. Spiritual needs of patients with cancer and family caregivers. Cancer Nursing. 2003;26:4, 260–66.

[16] Bilge A. Beliefs toward mental illness scale's validity and reliability study (in Turkish). Psikiyatri Hemsireliği AD Doktora Tezi, Ege Üniversitesi Sağlık Bilimleri Enstitüsü. 2006 İzmir.

[17] Çam O, Bilge A. Attitudes, beliefs toward mental illness (in Turkish). Anadolu Psikiyatri Dergisi. 2007;8:215–23.

[18] Demir N. Some philosophical opinions about human being (in Turkish). Felsefe Dünyası. 2004;40(2):77–93.

[19] Ulu M. Accordıng to James W. Fowler faith and structural pattern of faith (in Turkish). Bilimname Xxv, 2013/2. p. 157–68

[20] Sülü E. Spiritual care requirements of the mothers of the hospitalized children in intensive care units (in Turkish). Hemsirelik Programı Yüksek Lisans Tezi, Ege Üniversitesi Sağlık Bilimleri Enstitüsü. İzmir; 2006.

[21] Peter C. Hıll, Kenneth I. Pargament, Ralph W. Hood Jr, Michael E. Mccullough, James P. Swyers, David B. Larson, Brian J. Zınnbauer. Trans: Dr. Nurten Kimter, Din ve Maneviyatı Kavramlastırma: Birlesme ve Ayrılma Noktaları, Çanakkale Onsekiz Mart Üniversitesi İlahiyat Fakültesi Dergisi. 2013;3:85–118

[22] Religious Life Survey in Turkey, Presidency of Religious Affairs, Ankara; 2014.

[23] McCormick T.R. Spirituality and medicine (April 2014). https://depts.washington.edu/bioethx/topics/spirit.html [Accessed: 2016.08.06].

[24] https://humanism.org.uk/campaigns/religion-and-belief-some-surveys-and-statistics/ [Accessed: 2016.08.04].

[25] Carpenito LJ. Nursing diagnosis handbook (in Turkish). (Trans: F Erdemir). İstanbul: Nobel Tıp Kitabevleri; 2005.

[26] Baldacchino D. Spiritual care: is it the nurse's role? Spiritual Health Int. 2008;9(4):270–84. doi:10.1002/shi.363

[27] Wong KF, Lee LYK, Lee JKL, (2008) Hong Kong enrolled nurses' perceptions of spirituality and spiritual care. Int Nursing Rev. 2008;55:333–40. doi:10.1111/j.1466-7657.2008.00619.x

[28] Puchalski CM. The role of spirituality in health care. BUMC Proc. 2001;14:352–357.

[29] Koenig HG. Religion, spirituality, and medicine: research findings and implications for clinical practice. South Med J. 2004;97(12):1194–99.

[30] Pargament KI, Koenig HG, et al. Religious coping methods as predictors of psychological, physical and spiritual outcomes among medically ill elderly patients: a two-year longitudinal study. J Health Psychol. 2004;9:713. doi:10.1177/1359105304045366

[31] Pargament KI, Koenig HG, Tarakeshwar N, Hahn J. Religious struggle as a predictor of mortality among medically ill elderly patients. Arch Intern Med. 2001;161:1881–5. doi:10.1001/archinte.161.15.1881

[32] Vanderpool HY, Levin JS. Religion and medicine: how are they related? J Religion Health. 1990;29:9–17. doi:10.1007/BF00987090

[33] Puchalski C, Ferrell B, Virani R, Otis-Green S, Baird, P, Bull, J, Chochinov H, Handzo G, Nelson-Becker H, Prince-Paul M, Pugliese K, Sulmasy D. Improving the quality of spiritual care as a dimension of palliative care: the report of the consensus conference. J Palliat Med. 2009;12(10):885–904. doi:10.1089/jpm.2009.0142

[34] Ai A. Spiritual and religious involvement related to end-of-life decision-making in patients undergoing coronary by-pass graft surgery. Int J Psychiatry Med. 2008;38(1): 111–130. doi:10.2190/PM.38.1.k

[35] Anandarajah G, Hight E. Spirituality and medical practice: using the HOPE questions as a practical tool for spiritual assessment. Am Fam Physician. 2001:81–88.

[36] Dedeli Ö, Karadeniz G. An integrated psychosocial-spiritual model for cancer pain management (in Turkish). AĞRI. 2009;21(2):45–53.

[37] Harrington A. God and health: what more is there to say? Digital accsess to scolarship at Harvard. 2010. p. 1–27.

[38] Coyle J. Spirituality and health: towards a framework for exploring the relationship between spirituality and health. J Adv Nursing. 2002;37 (6):589–97. doi:10.1046/j.1365-2648.2002.02133.x

[39] Hall J. Making sense of spirituality, spirituality at the beginning of life. J Clin Nursing. 2006;15:804–10. doi:10.1111/j.1365-2702.2006.01650.x

[40] Strang S, Strang P, Ternestedt B. Spiritual needs as defined by Swedish nursing staff. J Clin Nursing. 2002;11:48–57. doi:10.1046/j.1365-2702.2002.00569.x

[41] Khorshid L, Arslan GG. Nursing and spiritual care. Ege Üniversitesi Hemsirelik Yüksek Okulu Dergisi. 2006;22(1):233–43. http://dergipark.ulakbim.gov.tr/egehemsire/article/download/5000152210/5000137999Benzer.

[42] Puchalski CM. Spirituality in the cancer trajectory. Ann Oncol. 2012;23 (3):49–55. doi: 10.1093/annonc/mds088

[43] Balboni TA, Vanderwerker LC, Block SD, Paulk ME, et al. Religiousness and spiritual support among advanced cancer patients and associations with end-of-life treatment preferences and quality of life. J Clin Oncol. 2007;25:555–60. doi:10.1200/JCO.2006.07.9046

[44] Hampton DM, Hollis DE, Lloyd DA, Taylor J, et al. Spiritual needs of persons with advanced cancer. Am J Hosp Palliat Care. 2007;24:42–8. doi:10.1177/1049909106295773

[45] Hsiao SM, Gau ML, Ingleton C, Ryan T, et al. An exploration of spiritual needs of Taiwanese patients with advanced cancer during the therapeutic processes. J Clin Nurs 2011;20:950–9. doi:10.1111/j.1365-2702.2010.03278.x

[46] Lin HR, Bauer-Wu SM. Psycho-spiritual well-being in patients with advanced cancer: an integrative review of the literature. J Adv Nurs. 2003;44:69–80.

[47] Sherman AC, Plante TG, Simonton S, Latif U, Anaissie EJ. Prospective study of religious coping among patients undergoing autologous stem cell transplantation. J Behav Med. 2009:118–128.

[48] Handzo, G, HG Koenig. Spiritual care: whose job is it anyway? Southern Medical Association, 2004. doi:10.1097/01.SMJ.0000146490.49723.AE

[49] Kavas E, Kavas N. Determination of the spiritual support perception of doctors, midwives and nurses about the need of spiritual care of the parents: Denizli sample (in Turkish). Turkish Stud Int Period Lang Lit Hist Turkish Or Turkic. 2015;10:449–60.

[50] Yılmaz M. Okyay N. Views related to spiritual care and spirituality of nurses (in Turkish). HEMAR-G 2009;3:41–52.

[51] Çelik AS, Özdemir F, Durmaz H, Pasinlioğlu T. Determining the perception level of nurses regarding spirituality and spiritual care and the factors that affect their perception level (in Turkish). Hacettepe Üniversitesi Hemsirelik Fakültesi Dergisi. 2014;1–12.

[52] http://www.diyanet.gov.tr/tr/icerik/hastanelerde-manevi-destek-donemi-basliyor %E2%80%A6/25477 [Accessed: 2016.08.01].

[53] Fortin AH, Barnett KG. Medical school curricula in spirituality and medicine. JAMA. 2004; 291(23): 2883. doi:10.1001/jama.291.23.2883

Chapter 7

The Veterans Affairs Patient Aligned Care Team (VA PACT), a New Benchmark for Patient-Centered Medical Home Models: A Review and Discussion

Balmatee Bidassie

Additional information is available at the end of the chapter

http://dx.doi.org/10.5772/66415

Abstract

Objective: Conduct a literature review on existing patient-centered medical home (PCMH) models and outline the differences and contributions.

Data sources: Systematic PCMH review data from PubMed database, from January 2000 to March 2013.

Results: Forty-eight (48) papers on various PCMH were included in the analysis. The types of collaborative PCMH models were compared in accordance to the scope of current PCMH demonstration projects, patient types, implementation strategy, and cross-functional team recruiting. The performance measurement tools and methods for data collection/analysis were thoroughly explored. Finally, the outcomes from PCMH models were evaluated in regard to patient experience, staff experience, quality of care, and economic outcomes.

Limitations: This review excluded the collaborative models which are not patient centered or patient oriented.

Conclusions and implications: Healthcare systems and their primary care practices are redesigning to achieve goals identified in PCMH models. However, implementation of these models requires major transformation. The Department of Veterans Affairs (VA) PCMH model, Patient Aligned Care Teams (PACT) model, has improved patients' and staff experience and care processes. PACT also includes innovative resources and tools to help healthcare teams develop a systematic approach to data-driven decision-making in healthcare transformation and should be considered when benchmarking for future PCMH model planning.

Keywords: collaborative care, patient-centered medical home, healthcare business process, Veterans Affairs, PACT

1. Introduction

The healthcare industry is driven to provide every patient with the best health care possible [1]. To reach this goal, provider organizations and third-party payers in healthcare facilities are implementing a variety of innovative high-quality programs in areas such as primary care [2–4], mobile health [5], and family care [6]. Although these sophisticated services provide invaluable resources for patients, in many cases they operate as silos, therefore, sometimes creating a complicated web of separate services which patients have to decipher. The patient-centered medical home (PCMH) is intended as a systematic approach for organizing primary care to coordinate and integrate healthcare services to provide a seamless platform of high-quality care considering the full spectrum of a patients' healthcare needs, with the goal to enhance patients' experiences [7, 8]. The term "home" is meant to describe friendly, accessible, personal, and supportive health care which is provided by one healthcare team and through the coordination of care when needed [9].

Currently, a variety of healthcare facilities and organizations have implemented different types of PCMH models [10–12]. Although there are several review papers that summarize the current design of PCMH models, implementation strategies, and latest evaluation results from pilot PCMH models [7, 13, 14], some topics are not discussed, such as the design of measurement tools to track the performance of PCMH implementation and the composition of PCMH teams. It was found that the Department of Veterans Affairs (VA), Veterans Health Administration (VHA) PCMH model, called Patient Aligned Care Team (PACT) model [15–17], includes innovative resources and tools to contribute to healthcare teams planning to develop a systematic approach to data-driven decision-making in healthcare transformation for future PCMH model. Integral to the success of the PACT model was the PACT Collaborative, which aided implementation.

The goal of this chapter is to systematically review the existing designs of typical PCMH models, such as the scope of PCMH projects and implementation strategies, examine process monitoring and measurement tools, and outcomes from quality of care measures such as patient satisfaction and staff efficiency. In addition, the author will outline VHA's realistic transformation opportunities and challenges in implementing PACT into their integrated healthcare systems on a national scale using the PACT Collaborative. The author will give examples of lessons learned by researchers, clinical staff, and policy partners during the early stages of PACT implementation which will be informative to other managed care or Accountable Care Organizations (ACOs) engaged in implementing PCMH models and may serve as a guideline to develop suitable models and implementation strategies for different healthcare organizations.

2. Review methods

This review conforms to the Preferred Reporting Items for Systematic Reviews and Meta-Analyses (PRISMA) standards [18]. An electronic search was conducted through the PubMed database for papers relative to the PCMH model and collaborative healthcare models published from January 2000 to March 2013. The search strategy used the text keywords for patient centered or medical home and related concepts for eligible study designs. The included studies were published in English and indexed from database inception. The exact search strings are listed in **Table 1**, and details of the number of articles in each category are listed in **Table 2**. This search found 1559 articles published during this time period.

The titles and abstracts obtained from the electronic search were screened by reviewers independently to eliminate duplicates and exclude articles not related to PCMH models and those that are not based on patient centered or medical home models. A full-text review was

Collaborative model design	Key components
	Customer population
	Disease type
	Improvement model
	Learning session
	Action period
	Sustainability
	Industrial engineer
Measurement tools/data analysis method	Change package
	Measurement tool
	Process mapping
	Voice of customer
	Information technology
	Electronic record
Outcomes	Care collaboration
	Access management
	Practice redesign
	Care integration
	Hospital utilization
	Patient satisfaction
	Quality of care
	Chronic disease
	Team communication
	Process efficiency
	Cost savings

Table 1. Search terms used for article search.

	Number of articles	
Search term	1/1/2000 to present	2010 to present
Patient-centered medical home model	1559	569
Measurement tool	8	3
Information technology	618	199
Improvement model	179	66
Learning session	15	1
Action period	11	0
Sustainability	48	14
Voice of customer	2	0
Care collaboration	172	71
Access management	108	54
Practice redesign	25	15
Team communication	94	37
Chronic disease	170	73
Model design	247	101
Electronic record	39	20
Hospital utilization	54	18
Patient satisfaction	270	85
Quality of care	587	248
Care integration	101	45
Industrial engineer	0	0
Change package	1	0
Process efficiency	25	5
Cost savings	26	12

Table 2. Number of articles in each category.

performed on the remaining articles, and abstracts were selected for inclusion in this review based on the following specified criteria: (1) All the articles should be peer-reviewed; (2) All interventions should meet the definition of PCMH defined by Agency for Healthcare Research and Quality (AHRQ) [19]; and (3) Outcome evaluations should be data-driven and generated from practical implementation of the PCMH model. Since it was found that there was a lack of consistent definitions and nomenclature for PCMH, a manual reference review of relevant review articles was conducted and an additional four papers were identified. Overall, the search process resulted in a total of 48 articles in the final systematic review. The article selection process is shown in **Figure 1**.

Based on the approach described in AHRQ's "Methods Guide for Effectiveness and Comparative Effectiveness Reviews" [20], each paper was evaluated independently by two

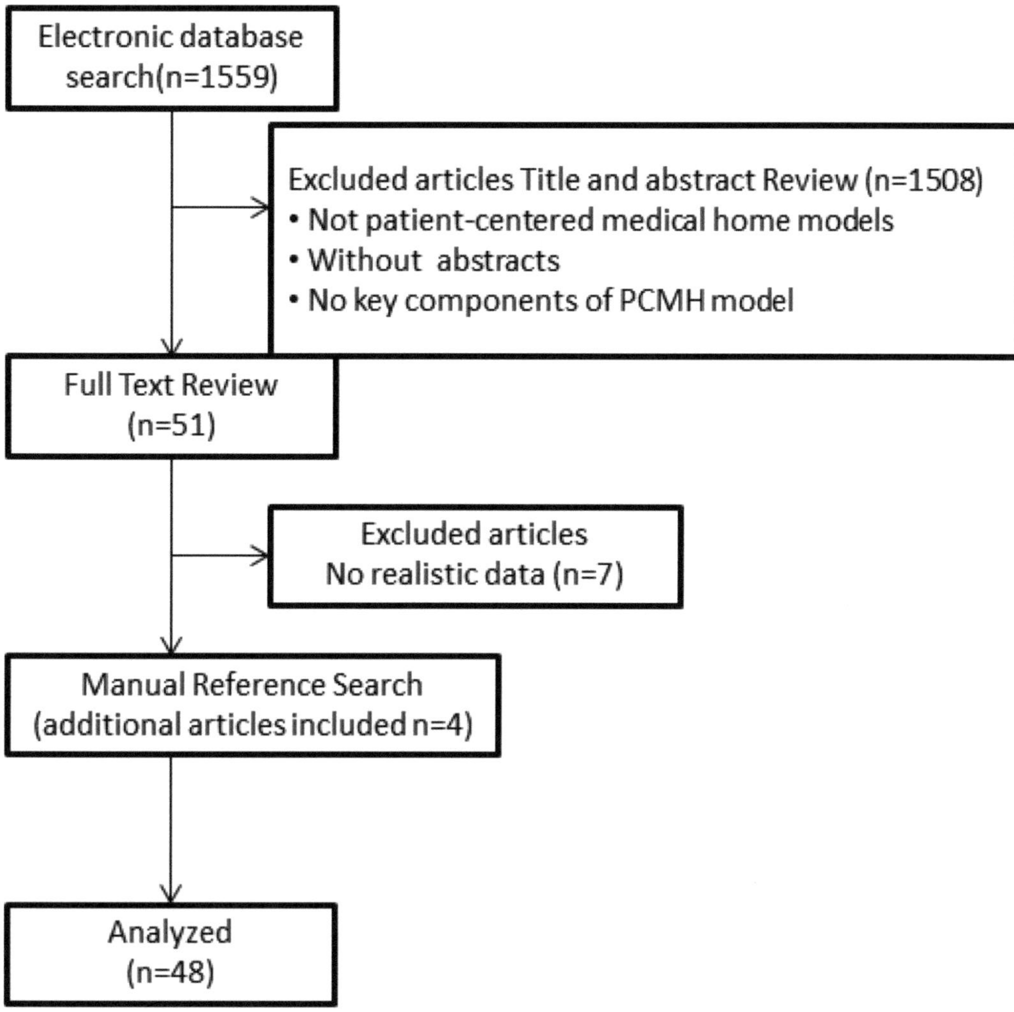

Figure 1. PCMH model article search results.

reviewers. Using the predefined criteria for methodological quality and adequacy of reporting for each study type, the quality of the study was judged in three levels: good, fair, or poor. Results of interest examined for PCMH effectiveness included key model components, data collection and analysis methods, performance measurement tools, quality improvement processes, care collaboration, and cost savings.

2.1. Review findings

2.1.1. PCMH scope and implementation strategies

As a new delivery model for primary care, the PCMH model provides comprehensive and coordinated care [21–23]. Systematic review results revealed various PCMH models are widely designed and verified by research institutes [17, 19], healthcare organizations [9, 24], clinical physicians [25–27], and other stakeholders [28–30]. Although most of the PCMH models share a similar mission to provide patient centered, comprehensive, and accessible care [31], there is substantial diversity not only in the scope of PCMH demonstration projects and patient types, but also in the implementation strategy at pilot sites.

Most of the PCMH models are natural extensions of overall healthcare management or area-wide quality improvement initiatives. For example, the PACT model focuses on access, care coordination and management, and practice redesign for primary care, which covers patient access [32, 33], healthcare business process redesign, and care organization problems. However, some models only focus on specific types of diseases. For example, chronic care collaborative models require long-term cooperation among cross-functional members [34–38]. Typical diseases of interest for chronic care collaborative include diabetes [39, 40] and cardiovascular diseases [41]. Furthermore, the complexity level of each disease is a vital factor for PCMH model design in these cases [42]. For those PCMH models which are developed to improve complex diseases, such as cancer care [43], it is important to enhance seamless cooperation among specialists [44, 45], primary physicians, nurses [29], pharmacists [46], and social workers [47].

There are also considerations for implementing PCMH models to focus on other subsets of the population, such as women. For PACT model, this is certainly a worthy area of focus as women now represent the fastest growing segment of new VA users [48]. Women tend to also have complex healthcare needs, which may affect how VA care is organized, providers are trained, and how the VA can best deliver gender-sensitive primary care.

Implementation strategies vary widely across each healthcare system. Although each PCMH model has its unique objectives, a high-functioning interdisciplinary primary care teams are required as a critical component of the patient-centered medical home for them to collaborate. A core feature of PACT which showed huge promise for improving primary care at the VA was the creation of teamlets (small teams). A PACT teamlet required reorganization of primary care personnel into assumed new roles. It is a primary care team that generally consists of a primary care provider (MD, NP, PA), registered nurse care manager, clinical associate (LPN or medical assistant/health technician), an administrative associate (MA/MSA/health technician), and pharmacists, and they are integrated to provide on-site, in-office coordinated care [28, 30, 49]. The transformation into this team-based approach requires the following: (1) ensuring adequate staffing in all team roles, (2) devoting resources to in-depth training for all employees in communication and other skills needed to maximize team success, and (3) aligning the broader hospital system with PCMH decentralized, team-based approach [50, 51].

Team-based model is a fundamental shift in the roles and relationships among clinical personnel. Therefore, it creates a need for a more nuanced team-based audit, since currently the ownership of clinical performance still rests largely with the provider, despite the move to more team-based health care [52]. The team-based model can also create an opportunity to mitigate any discontinuity of care due to residency transitions [53].

During the beginning stages of strategic planning for implementing VA's PACT, top challenges faced by primary care directors were reviewed and included clinical informatics, chronic pain management, and care coordination [54]. In the early stages of implementation, several challenges were identified to move to the team-based approach including: (1) short-staffing undermined development of team-based working relationships; (2) lack of co-location of PACT members in clinic and difficulty communicating with residents when they were off-site hampered communication and; (3) limited clinic hours of part-time primary care providers and residents prevented clinicians to get the training and reinforcement of PCMH principles which delayed the team formation [55].

Considering the many challenges to transitioning to a team-based approach, PACT's implementation strategy consists of various supportive initiatives including a national face-to-face kickoff conference, American College of Physicians (ACP) Medical Home Builder survey, the Centers of Excellence learning centers, national conference calls, common metrics, and the PACT Collaborative [17].

Some non-VA PCMH models use similar steps as the PACT, whereas others used the following: (1) emphasizing the role of nurses in educating patients [56], (2) PCMH principles based on complexity, care-coordination activities, and techniques to measure family satisfaction [57], (3) patient-centered care plan (PCCP) document to enhance care for complex patients and change the relationships with health team members [58], and (4) the adoption of PDSA cycles in PCMH implementation in large primary care and multi-specialty medical groups [27].

Communication among multiple stakeholders is regarded as one of the key factors to ensure high quality of care. PCMH projects normally involve cooperation of multiple stakeholders and some of the reported key communication barriers for clinicians when performing across-discipline consultations include as follows: (1) lack of effective standardized communication processes, (2) practice style differences, and (3) inadequate PC training [59]. Sharing of real-time information on the status and results of PCMH projects and integrating the instant feedback into decision-making are two key factors that contributed to the final achievement of each PCMH-based project. Multiple supportive technologies and methods are deployed to facilitate communication, such as conference calls, electronic communication, and group e-mails [9, 17]. In addition to these tools, PACT utilizes the Microsoft SharePoint™ platform to share all real-time information which records all the updates with version tracking of supporting documentation [9]. In addition, the collaborative initiative within PACT adapted the Institute for Healthcare Improvement (IHI) Breakthrough Series Collaborative model [60], to deploy a web-based communication platform to train team members (similar to an e-learning system) and web-based storyboards for teams to review the results [61]. Within PACT, there is also a "toolkit" used at VA facilities nationwide to support teams to share, download, and adopt information in order to more effectively implement PCMH principles and improve local performance on VA metrics [62]. The toolkit is an online repository of ready-to-use tools created by VA staff (physicians, nurses, and other team members). PACT team member perspectives on the toolkit ranged from enthusiastic to not having time to review the contents of the toolkit.

2.1.2. *Performance monitoring systems*

While PACT Collaborative utilizes "PACT Compass" metrics [63] from VHA's information systems to organized broad domains, such as access, coordination of care, and continuity, most other PCMH implementation strategies dedicate considerable resources to direct practice support by helping the teams reorganize workflows and provide tools to enhance practice capacity. A Physicians Practice Connection-PCMH (PPC-PCMH) model categorizes the principles into different levels based on their priorities and gives a numeric score of 0–24 points to the performance [64]. Some measurement tools are web-based with data automatically collected by Health Information Technology (HIT) systems [65], such as electronic medical records [66, 67]. The traditional ways of data collection, such as direct observation [68], patient interview, internal survey [58, 69], and audio recording [33], are used to collect information about patients' opinions.

Monthly and annual reports are utilized to track performance improvement and to compare the practice results of PCMH models. Some PCMH models invite clinical staff, such as physicians, to summarize the results of the medical treatment improvement by adopting the PCMH model [68]. In the PACT Collaborative, 250 medical teams from five regions were required to submit monthly performance reports to record a core set of metrics that assessed the program's impact on access, continuity of care, patient engagement and satisfaction, panel management, coordination of care, and clinical improvement [17].

Voice of customer (VOC) analysis is a useful tool to collect information about the current state of the healthcare business process, identify the potential problems, define the overall improvement goals, and test the acceptance rate of PCMH model by end users. Several projects use customer surveys to gather data from multiple stakeholders and analyzed the results by some statistical algorithms, such as regression modeling and standard ordinary least squares [70]. As of March 2012, Veterans Affairs include questions in the Survey of Healthcare Experience of Patients (SHEP) [71] to help understand the Veterans' satisfaction with VHA ambulatory care and to support assessment of VA's initiative to provide Veteran-centered primary care through the implementation of PACT.

While the use of relevant performance measures is an effective guide for quality improvement in PCMH models, there is little information in the literature on staff perceptions of performance metric implementation in these PCMH settings. Based on research conducted in PACT, it was found that primary care staff perceived performance metrics as time-consuming and not consistently aligned with PACT principles of care. Also, they found that metrics were as follows: (1) not reflecting Veteran's priorities, (2) represented an opportunity cost, (3) implemented with little communication or transparency, and (4) not well-adapted to team-based care. Based on this, it appears that there are gaps between the theory and reality of performance metric implementation, and these gaps should be considered when implementing a PCMH [72].

2.1.3. Outcomes from PCMH models

Quality of care is considered one of the most important indicators to judge the effects of new process improvement models. Christensen et al. [73] verified that the Walter Reed PCMH had reduced costs while at least maintaining, if not improving, access to and quality of care, and to determine whether access, quality, and cost impacts differed by chronic condition status. Henderson et al. [74] discussed the guiding principles of PCMH model to improve quality of care and demonstrated these principles with a case study from the experience of a care coordinator in a rural PCMH in Maine. Rosenberg et al. [75] reported on the experience of

University of Pennsylvania Medical Center Health Plan as part of a large, integrated delivery and financing system of PCMH to improve access to high-quality care for more Americans at a lower cost.

PCMH models have the goal of improving the patients' satisfaction and staff efficiency. Access management is one of the vital aspects that affected patient satisfaction. True et al. [22], identified successful strategies used by early adopters to overcome barriers to change the access management, which might increase patient satisfaction. Segel et al. [76] demonstrated that the patient-centered collaborative care model could improve discharge efficiency, staff communication, and patient satisfaction. However, the relative research to verify the performance improvement of medical staff members is lacking in comparison with the research that explored patient satisfaction. The patient satisfaction survey in the PACT model (SHEP) supported positive outcomes of patient access improvement [71]. Jaen et al. [32] evaluated patient relative outcomes, which included satisfaction with service relationship after implementing the PCMH model for more than 2 years.

2.1.4. Economics outcomes from PCMH models

PCMH models have the potential to reduce costs [77] and create optimal strategies for healthcare utilization. Based on the selected articles, the cost reduction analysis mainly focuses on emergency department utilization, inpatient admissions, and total costs. Adoption of the PCMH model has been shown to reduce patient waiting time, improve access to care, and reduce inappropriate emergency room care [78, 79, 80], especially for the elder group of patients. Domino et al. [81] described a case study to show the decrease in emergency department utilization for children with chronic and serious diseases. It is the intention of the VA to evaluate the impact of the medical home on admissions and emergency department use, both of which may serve as proxies for cost [17]. Although the cost among PCMH patients was significant in the first few years and may be higher than non-PCMH patients considering the project cost [82], the expected projected reduction of cost of the PCMH model as the project is extended more long term is not discussed in detail within the articles.

3. Benchmarking VA PCMH model—PACT

In 2010, VHA (the largest integrated healthcare system in the United States, serving more than 8 million veterans) launched PACT (a national implementation of a PCMH model) to transform primary care delivery by improving the delivery of patient-centered care. PACT's aim to improve access, continuity, coordination, and comprehensiveness using team-based care that is patient driven and patient centered [83]. This national rollout of PCMH to all VA primary care practices in more than 150 medical centers and over 800 community-based outpatient clinics (in 900 primary care clinics nationwide, with 120 located in academically affiliated medical centers) aimed to offer accessible, comprehensive, and seamless care for meeting the customized needs and expectations of each Veteran [9, 84]. As a result, over 7000 primary care teams across the nation are in the process of transforming their operations.

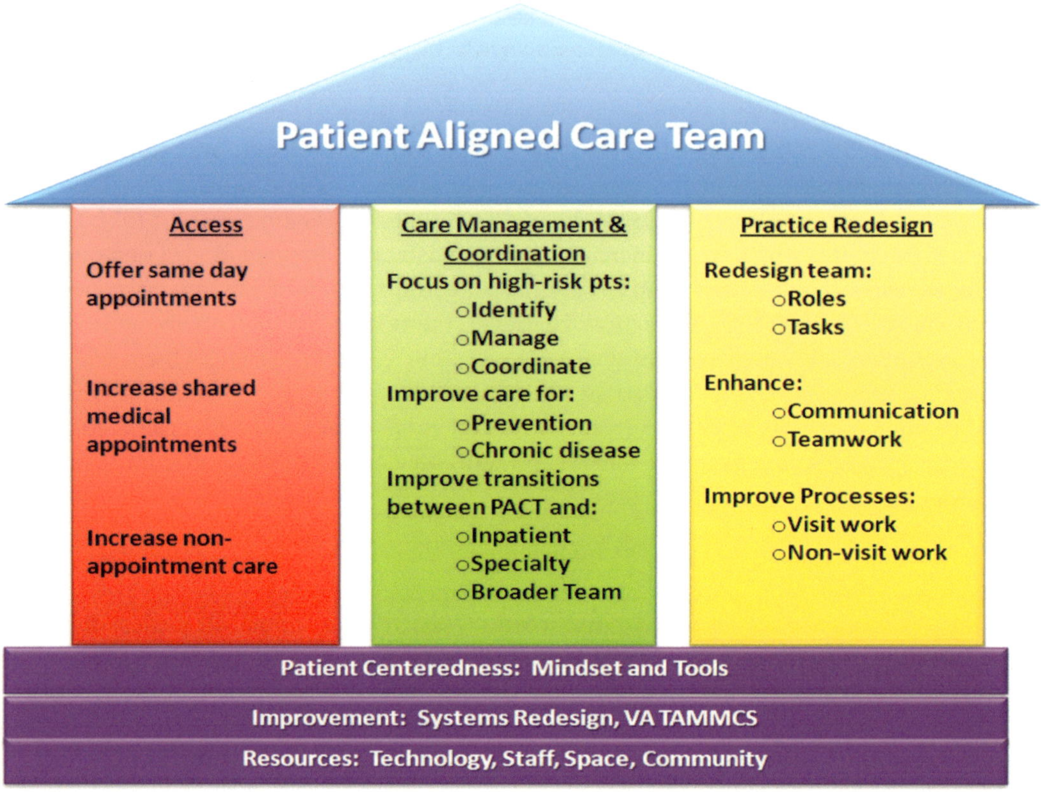

Figure 2. PACT three-pillar model. Reproduced with permission [85].

The PACT model (**Figure 2**) was designed to translate the PCMH model's symbolic vision of a "home" into a tangible implementation plan where the roof and overarching goal are patient centeredness. The foundation of the home includes critical resources and the use of process improvement methodologies such as LEAN [85]. The three pillars of the PACT model are access, care management and coordination, and practice redesign. Each pillar represents a vital content area necessary to achieve a true patient-centered medical home and includes several primary and supporting measures to record the progress on each aim, summarized in Appendix 1.

VHA facilities that were most successful in implementation of the overarching goals have an internal capability for organizational learning and development [86], and deployable evidence-based quality improvement strategies that give teams the tools needed to adjust structures and processes to meet their goals [87]. In addition to the individual efforts being conducted at each facility, VHA used a collaborative learning model, PACT Collaborative [88], as a key approach to disseminate PACT concepts and changes, with the intention to successfully support the implementation goals of the PACT model in each facility.

The PACT Collaborative is a learning environment based on the IHI Breakthrough Series Collaborative model [89] (**Figure 3**). **Figure 4** illustrates the modifications, which are the addition of VHA national process improvement TAMMCS (vision, analysis, team, aim, map,

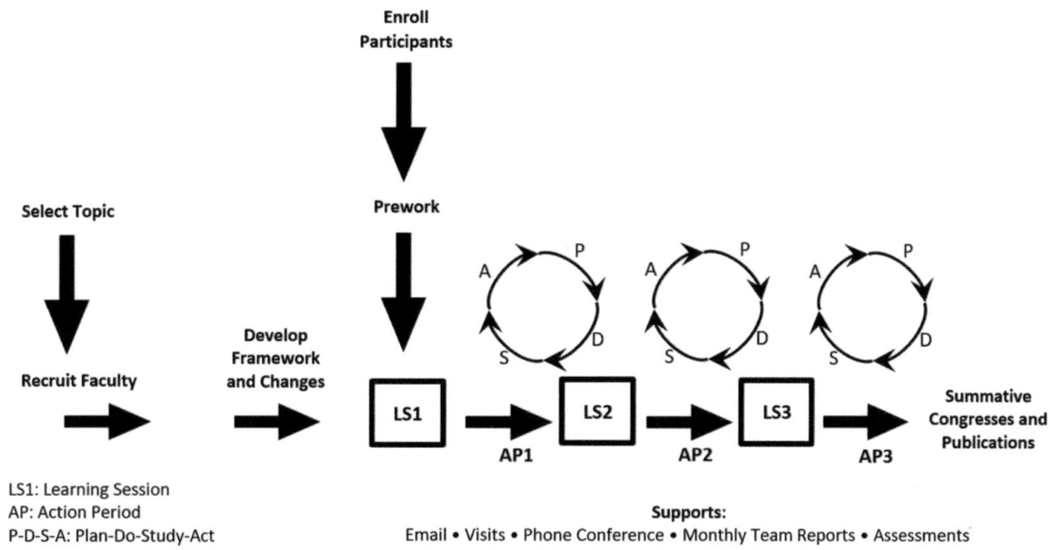

Figure 3. Institute for Healthcare Improvement (IHI) Breakthrough Series Collaborative Model.

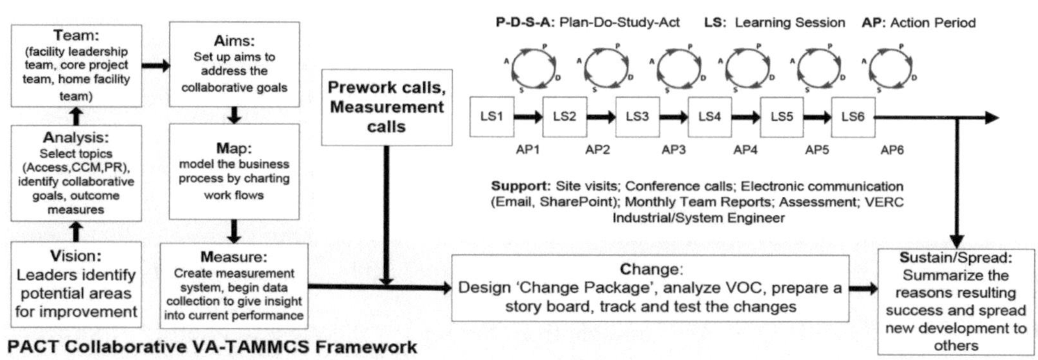

Figure 4. PACT three-pillar model. Reproduced with permission [85]

measure, change, and sustain) along with the inclusion of 3 additional learning sessions [90] (**Figure 4**).

The PACT Collaborative model was made up of five regional PACT Collaborative and approximately 250–350 individuals from 141 teams participated in six face-to-face learning sessions across 21 months, where learning sessions were adopted for exchanging ideas through peer-to-peer meetings and audio conferences, and training a sample of patients or caregivers from patients' families with basic and necessary medical information. In each of the regions, there were industrial engineers (IEs) and coordinators from the Veterans Engineering Resource Centers to serve as coaching, teaching, and process improvement experts to collect data, track improvement progress, and make process improvement decisions [88]. This novel addition to the program brought an unparalleled level of quality improvement expertise. Their work involved problem analysis, aim definition, team creation, principle and measurement tool design, performance improvement with the combination of learning sessions and action periods, and Plan-Do-Study-Act (PDSA) [91] cycles.

Within the PACT Collaborative, Excel-based measurement tools, PACT Compass (a consolidated combination of care quality measures) was used to track the overall PACT PCMH model from the national level to provide system-wide sharing of data and allowing performance improvement to be monitored at the team level [92]. The performance measures in the collaborative were as follows: (1) PACT Collaborative participant surveys; (2) Coach Assessment Scores and Plan-Do-Study-Act (PDSA) data; and (3) PACT Compass (national measures to assess PACT implementation within VA healthcare system). At the end of the collaborative, most participants reported the PACT Collaborative was needed to implement PACT. Team members reported that involvement of the industrial engineers, use of the measurement tools, the change packages, and monthly reports improved teams' performance from all perspectives related to access, care coordination, and knowledge gains by the teams [88]. Over 80% of the teams were successful in process improvement initiatives that increased the number of same-day appointments, increasing non-face-to-face care, and improving team communication [87].

4. Discussion

Based on the results of the review, there is a significant opportunity to document the progress of PCMH projects and identify standard performance measurement indicators for PCMH models. If more standard performance measurement indicators are identified and used, future meta-analyses could be performed to distinguish the effects of the PCMH models in comparison with non-PCMH models or current practices. The PACT model, utilizing the PACT Collaborative, can serve as a guideline to develop suitable models and implementation strategies that include evaluation tools inherent to a successful PCMH model for healthcare organizations.

The PACT model and a few other models from the review mentioned monthly reports and documentation to track the status of PCMH projects; however, there was no standard format for reports and many evaluations are not documented well enough to demonstrate the results of models, and often those that are documented can only identify non-generalizable outcomes [93]. The PACT model is unique in that the PACT Collaborative heavily utilized industrial engineers in partnership with clinicians as part of the core planning and project team to review monthly reports, analyze the results, and assist the faculty for further improvement suggestions. By employing such strategies as process mapping, VOC analysis, PDSA cycles, and a variety of communication techniques, the PACT model was able to document their progress and improve outcomes. Other PCMH models have had difficulty in implementation due to a lack of staff trained in the implementation methods and the burden of data collection [94].

Although the articles in this review did not uncover cost reductions associated with PCMH, recent research has discovered the actual cost savings occur once full implementation, versus partial implementation, of the model has been actualized [95]. To ensure the implementation results and improvement of quality care and collaboration efficiency, all stakeholders should have assessment methods to evaluate the performance and a road map to guide them to implement customized PCMH models into their facilities successfully. Data collection and analysis are important elements to summarize the achievements from previous steps, identify the valuable stories to share with other groups, and sustain the results to broader adoption fields. However, there is a need for a comprehensive theory to select key indicators which could evaluate the PCMH model. In addition, more efficient technologies to share and integrate real-time information about collaborative procedures are needed.

While PACT primary care personnel viewed PACT positively as a model, they reported insufficient staffing and low-functioning team members as barriers to achieve highly functioning teamlets [96]. In response to this, the PACT Collaborative could resolve these barriers with evaluation tools and team member training, as one study confirmed the Collaborative enabled care teams to achieve over 80% of their aims, increased the number of PDSAs through implementation to 93%, and was deemed necessary to implement PACT [88]. Additionally, team process and effectiveness measures had stronger associations with perceived improvements in teams' abilities to deliver patient-centered care [97].

The collaborative learning model may also be an effective way to leverage a small number of staff and personnel across a large patient population [88]. As such, specialty-care clinics could be converted to function as a PCMH as these clinics often continue to operate as silos within a large, integrated healthcare system and are still functioning with a wide variation in patients' receipt of care [98]. Overall, the VA's PACT model, and particularly the PACT Collaborative within this model, addresses many of the obstacles PCMH models face from implementation to evaluation and may serve as a benchmark for future PCMH planning in order to enhance future models.

5. Conclusions

A limitation of this review is that it excluded the collaborative models which are not patient centered or patient oriented. In the future, it could be an interesting area of research to compare similarities between models which are patient centered and those which are not patient centered.

More research should also focus on the added patient values and return-on-investment of the PCMH models, particularly over a longer course of time. Another possible area for future research would be to build upon health information technology (HIT), such as electronic health record and electronic identification which could streamline the process of information exchange, and increase the patient's access to health services. Although the current HIT can support many of the core principles of PCMH, it does not have all the functionalities to facilitate the model directly, which might be a potential research focus for healthcare-IT specialists.

In summary, the PCMH model has been recognized as a promising solution to supply patients with advanced primary care service. There is a large variety in the scope of current PCMH projects, as well as in the design, implementation, and evaluation of these projects. The PACT model is a large, successful example of a national PCMH project, and along with the PACT Collaborative, could serve as a standard for future PCMH models to reference when determining their designs, implementation strategies, and evaluation techniques.

Acknowledgements

The author would like to thank Xiaoyu Ma, PhD for assisting with the literature search and serving as a second reviewer along with the author. Thanks are also given to Amanda Kovach for her assistance editing and proofreading the manuscript.

Appendix

Aim	Primary measure	Supporting measure
Access	• Third next available appointment OR • Difference between desired date andactual appointment date • Percent of care provided outside of single provider appointment venues • Continuity • Percent of calls answered within 30 s • Percent of patient-generated e-mails responded within 24 h • Percent of care provided in group visits	• Panel size • Demand, supply and activity • No-show rate • Cancel and reschedule rate • Phone abandonment rate • First call problem resolution • Others as desired and needed • Group clinic stops • Average visit frequency
Practice Redesign	• Cycle time (and subsets) • Minutes behind • Ratio of red zone to total cycle time • Percent increase in teamlet huddles/week • Percent increase in team meetings/month • Pre- and post-team communication assessment	• % patients notified of test results within 7 days of test • % appointments started on time • % decrease in interruptions during the appointment • % refills done within 24 h • % forms completed/returned to patient within 72 hours
Care Coordination and Management	• Percent of high-risk patients being actively managed • Percent of patients with contact or visit within 48 hours/7 days of transition from ED or hospital • Percent adherence to PC portion of service agreement (right patient with correct work-up) • Percent increase in 2-way pre-discharge patient handoff communication	• Medication reconciliation rates on transitions (sample) • Laboratory reconciliation rates on transitions (sample) • Percent patients offered age appropriate preventative strategies and screening • Percent of patients by chronic disease active on a registry

Additional relevant measures

• Panel turnover rate • Length of primary care in dept • Panel DCG	• Octane (Specialty) • MHV-SM data • My HealtheVet enrollment • Patient complaint data	• RN/LPN/Clerk mix • Panel average age • Specialty referral rate

Appendix 1. Summary of the primary and supporting measures.

Author details

Balmatee Bidassie

Address all correspondence to: balmatee.bidassie@va.gov

VHA Office of Strategic Integration (OSI), Veterans Engineering Resource Center (VERC), Department of Veterans Affairs (VA), Center for Applied Systems Engineering (VA-CASE), Richard L. Roudebush Indianapolis VA Medical Center, Indianapolis, United States

References

[1] Healthcare Industry. [Online] Available from: http://en.wikipedia.org/wiki/Health_care_industry [Accessed: 2013-02-04].

[2] Michael M, Schaffer SD, Egan PL, Little BB, Pritchard PS. Improving wait times and patient satisfaction in primary care. J Healthc Qual. 2013; 35(2): 50–60.

[3] Coma E, Ferran M, Méndez L, Iglesias B, Fina F, et al. Creation of a synthetic indicator of quality of care as a clinical management standard in primary care. Springerplus. 2013; 2(1): 51.

[4] Brennan SE, Bosch M, Buchan H, Green SE. Measuring team factors thought to influence the success of quality improvement in primary care: a systematic review of instruments. Implement Sci. 2013; 8(1): 20.

[5] Källander K, Tibenderana JK, Akpogheneta OJ, Strachan DL, Hill Z, et al. Mobile health (mHealth) approaches and lessons for increased performance and retention of community health workers in low- and middle-income countries: a review. J Med Internet Res. 2013; 15(1): 17.

[6] Kuo DZ, Houtrow AJ, Arango P, Kuhlthau KA, Simmons JM, et al. Family-centered care: current applications and future directions in pediatric health care. Matern Child Health J. 2012; 16: 297–305.

[7] Jackson GL, Powers BJ, Chatterjee R, Bettger JP. The patient-centered medical home a systematic review. Ann Intern Med. 2012; 158(3): 169–97.

[8] Alexander JA, Cohen GR, Wise CG, Green LA. The policy context of patient centered medical homes: perspectives of primary care providers. J Gen Intern Med. 2013; 28(1): 147–53.

[9] VHA Systems Redesign Program Office, Patient Centered Medical Home Collaborative Prework Guide. 2010.

[10] Harbrecht MG, Latts LM. Colorado's patient-centered medical home pilot met numerous obstacles, yet saw results such as reduced hospital admissions. Health Affairs. 2012; 319: 2010–7.

[11] Maeng DD, Davis DE, Tomcavage J, Graf TR, Procopio KM. Improving patient experience by transforming primary care: evidence from Geisinger's patient-centered medical homes. Popul Health Manag. 2013;16(3): 157–63. Available from: http://online.liebertpub.com/doi/pdfplus/10.1089/pop.2012.0048 [Accessed 2013-02-26].

[12] Hudak RP, Julian R, Kugler J, Dorrance K, Lynch S, et al. The patient-centered medical home: a case study in transforming the military health system. Mil Med. 2013; 178(2): 146–52.

[13] Peikes D, Zutshi A, Genevro JL, Parchman ML, Meyers DS. Early evaluations of the medical home: building on a promising start. Am J Manag Care. 2012; 18(2): 105–22.

[14] Hoff T, Weller W, DePuccio M. The patient-centered medical home: a review of recent research. Med Care Res Rev. 2012; 69(6): 619–44.

[15] VHA Primary Care Program Office. Patient Aligned Care Team (PACT). Available from http://www.va.gov/primarycare/pact/ [Accessed 2013-02-06].

[16] Rosland A, Nelson K, Sun H, Dolan ED, Maynard C, Bryson C, Stark R, Shear JM, Kerr E, Fihn SD, Schectman G. The patient-centered medical home in Veterans Health Administration. Am J Manag Care. 2013; 19(7): 263–72.

[17] Klein S. The Veterans Health Administration: Implementing patient-centered medical homes in the nation's largest integrated delivery system. Commonwealth Fund. 2011; 16: 1537–60.

[18] Preferred Reporting Items for Systematic Reviews and Meta-Analyses. PRISMA statement. Available from: http://www.prisma-statement.org/ [Accessed 2013-02-08].

[19] Agency for Healthcare Research and Quality. What is the PCMH? AHRQ's definition of the medical home. Available from: http://pcmh.ahrq.gov/portal/server.pt/community/pcmhhome/1483/PCMHDefining%20the%20PCMH_v2 [Accessed 2013-03-11].

[20] Agency for Healthcare Research and Quality. Methods guide for effectiveness and comparative effectiveness review. Available at http://effectivehealthcare.ahrq.gov/index.cfm/search-for-guides-reviews-and-reports/?pageaction=displayproduct&productid=318 [Accessed 2013-02-14].

[21] Rittenhouse DR, Casalino LP, Gillies RR, Shortell SM, Lau B. Measuring the medical home infrastructure in large medical groups. Health Affairs. 2008; 27(5): 1246–58.

[22] True G, Butler AE, Lamparska BG, Lempa ML, Shea JA, et al. Open access in the patient-centered medical home: lessons from the veterans health administration. J Gen Intern Med. 2013; 28(4): 539–45.

[23] Takach M. About half of the states are implementing patient-centered medical homes for their Medicaid populations. Health Aff (Millwood). 2012; 31(11): 2432–40.

[24] Takane AK, Hunt SB. Transforming primary care practices in a Hawai'i Island clinic: obtaining patient perceptions on patient centered medical home. Hawaii J Med Public Health. 2012; 71(9): 253–8.

[25] Baxter L, Nash DB. Implementing the patient-centered medical home model for chronic disease care in small medical practices: practice group characteristics and physician understanding. Am J Med Qual. 2013; 28(2): 113–9.

[26] Rich EC, Lipson D, Libersky J, Peikes DN, Parchman ML. Organizing care for complex patients in the patient-centered medical home. Ann Fam Med. 2012; 10: 60–2.

[27] Rittenhouse DR, Casalino LP, Shortell SM, McClellan SR, Gillies RR, et al. Small and medium-size physician practices use few patient-centered medical home processes. Health Aff (Millwood). 2011; 30(8): 1575–84.

[28] Berdine HJ, Skomo ML. Development and integration of pharmacist clinical services into the patient-centered medical home. J Am Pharm Assoc. 2012; 52(5): 661–7.

[29] Tomcavage J, Littlewood D, Salek D, Sciandra J. Advancing the role of nursing in the medical home model. Nurs Adm Q. 2012; 36(3): 194–202.

[30] Haines SL, DeHart RM, Flynn AA, Hess KM, Marciniak MW, et al. Academic pharmacy and patient-centered health care: a model to prepare the next generation of pharmacists. J Am Pharm Assoc. 2011; 51(2): 194–202.

[31] Reid RJ, Fishman PA, Yu O, Ross TR, Tufano JT, et al. Patient-centered medical home demonstration: a prospective, quasi-experimental, before and after evaluation. Am J Manag Care. 2009; 15: 71–87.

[32] Jaén CR, Ferrer RL, Miller WL, Palmer RF, Wood R, et al. Patient outcomes at 26 months in the patient-centered medical home national demonstration project. Ann Fam Med. 2010; 8(1): 557–67.

[33] Bichel A, Erfle S, Wiebe V, Axelrod D, Conly J. Improving patient access to medical services: preventing the patient from being lost in translation. Healthc Q. 2009; 13: 61–8.

[34] Sidorov JE. The patient-centered medical home for chronic illness: is it ready for prime time? Health Aff. 2008; 27(5): 1231–4.

[35] Gabbay RA, Bailit MH, Mauger DT, Wagner EH, Siminerio L. Multipayer patient-centered medical home implementation guided by the chronic care model. Jt Comm J Qual Patient Saf. 2011; 37(6): 265–73.

[36] Ortiz G, Fromer L. Patient-centered medical home in chronic obstructive pulmonary disease. J Multidiscip Healthc. 2011; 4: 357–65.

[37] Gulley SP, Rasch EK, Chan L. If we build it, who will come? Working-age adults with chronic health care needs and the medical home. Med Care. 2011; 49(2): 149–55.

[38] Hennessey B, Suter P, Harrison G. The home-based chronic care model: a platform for partnership for the provision of a patient-centered medical home. Caring. 2010; 29(2): 18–24.

[39] Jortberg BT, Miller BF, Gabbay RA, Sparling K, Dickinson WP. Patient-centered medical home: how it affects psychosocial outcomes for diabetes. Curr Diab Rep. 2012; 12(6): 721–8.

[40] Johnson JA, Al Sayah F, Wozniak L, Rees S, Soprovich A, et al. Controlled trial of a collaborative primary care team model for patients with diabetes and depression: rationale and design for a comprehensive evaluation. BMC Health Serv Res. 2012; 12: 258–69.

[41] Hatzichristou D, Tsimtsiou Z. Prevention and management of cardiovascular disease and erectile dysfunction: toward a common patient-centered care model. Am J Cardiol. 2005; 96(12B): 80–4.

[42] Shippee ND, Shah ND, May CR, Mair FS, Montori VM. Cumulative complexity: a functional, patient-centered model of patient complexity can improve research and practice. J Clin Epidemiol. 2012; 65(10): 1041–51.

[43] Sarfaty M, Wender R, Smith R. Promoting cancer screening within the Patient Centered Medical Home. CA Cancer J Clin. 2011; 61(6): 397–408.

[44] Kirschner N, Barr MS. Specialists/subspecialists and the patient-centered medical home. Chest. 2010; 137(1): 200–4.

[45] O'Neill JL, Cunningham TL, Wiitala WL, and Bartley EP. Collaborative hypertension case management by Registered Nurses and Clinical Pharmacy Specialists within the Patient Aligned Care Teams (PACT) Model. J Gen Intern Med. 2014. 29(Suppl 2): S675 –81.

[46] Choe HM, Farris KB, Stevenson JG, Townsend K, Diez HL, et al. Patient-centered medical home: developing, expanding, and sustaining a role for pharmacists. Am J Health Syst Pharm. 2012; 69(12): 1063–71.

[47] Zimmerman J, Dabelko HI. Collaborative models of patient care: new opportunities for hospital social workers. Soc Work Health Care. 2007; 44(4): 33–47.

[48] Yano EM, Haskell S, Hayes P. Delivery of Gender-Sensitive Comprehensive Primary Care to Women Veterans: Implications for VA Patient Aligned Care Teams. J Gen Intern Med. 2013; 29(Suppl 2): S703–7.

[49] Dolovich L. Ontario pharmacists practicing in family health teams and the patient-centered medical home. Ann Pharmacother. 2012; 46(4): 33–9.

[50] Tuepker A, Kansagara D, Skaperdas E, Nicolaidis C, Joos C, Alperin M, Hickam D. "We've Not Gotten Even Close to What We Want to Do": a Qualitative Study of Early Patient-Centered Medical Home Implementation. J Gen Intern Med. 2014; 29(Suppl 2): S614–22.

[51] True G, Stewart GL, Lampman M, Pelak M, Solimeo SL. Teamwork and delegation in medical homes: primary care staff perspectives in the Veteran Health Administration. J Gen Intern Med. 2014; 29(Suppl 2): S632–9.

[52] Hysong S, Knox M, Haidet P. Examining Clinical Performance Feedback in Patient Aligned Care Teams. J Gen Intern Med. 2014; 29(Suppl 2): 667–74.

[53] Wang ES, Conde MV, Simon B, Leykum LK. Exploring End-of-Residency Transitions in a VA Patient Aligned Care Team. J Gen Intern Med. 2014; 29(Suppl 2): 649–58.

[54] Farmer MM, Rose DE, Rubenstein LV, Canelo IA, Schectman G, Stark R, Yano E. Challenges facing primary care practices aiming to implement patient-centered medical homes. J Gen Intern Med. 2014; 29(Suppl 2): S555–62.

[55] Forman J, Harrod M, Robinson C, Annis-Emeott A, Ott J, Saffar D, Krein S Greenstone C. First things first: foundational requirements for a medical home in an academic medical center. J Gen Intern Med. 2014; 29(Suppl 2): 640–648.

[56] Wood MR, Bolyard D. Making education count: the nurse's role in asthma education using a medical home model of care. J Pediatr Nurs. 2011; 26(6): 552–8.

[57] Cooley WC, McAllister JW. Building medical homes: improvement strategies in primary care for children with special health care needs. Pediatrics. 2004; 113(5):1499–506.

[58] Council LS, Geffken D, Valeras AB, Orzano AJ, Rechisky A, et al. A medical home: changing the way patients and teams relate through patient-centered care plans. Fam Syst Health. 2012; 30(3): 190–8.

[59] Chang ET, Wells KB, Young AS, Stockdale S, Johnson MD. The anatomy of primary care and mental health clinician communication: a quality improvement case study. J Gen Intern Med. 2013; 29(Suppl 2):S598–606.

[60] Institute for Healthcare Improvement. The Breakthrough Series: IHI's Assessment Scale for Collaborative. 2004.

[61] Boushon B, Provost L, Gagnon J, Carver P. Using a virtual breakthrough series collaborative to improve access in primary care. Jt Comm J Qual Patient Saf. 2006; 32(10): 573–84.

[62] Luck J, Bowman C, York L, Midboe A, Taylor T, et al. Multimethod evaluation of the VA's Peer-to-Peer Toolkit for patient-centered medical home implementation. J Gen Intern Med. 2014; 29(Suppl 2): S572–8.

[63] Medical Home Builder Survey VISN Detail. Available from: https://secure reports2.vssc.med.va.gov/ReportServer/Pages/ReportViewer.aspx?%2fPC%2fPC+Medical+Home%2fMainMenu&rs%3a-Command=Render [Accessed 2014-01-03].

[64] Mina L. Harkins. Introduction and overview: NCQA's PPC-PCMH recognition program. Available from http://www.cthealthpolicy.org/webinars/20100202_mharkins_ppc_pcmh.pdf [Accessed 2013-02-20].

[65] Miller C. Patient-centered medical home care model: IT considerations. MD Advis 2011; 4(4): 23–6.

[66] O'Malley AS, Cohen GR, Grossman JM. Electronic medical records and communication with patients and other clinicians: are we talking less? Issue Brief Cent Stud Health Syst Change. 2010 Apr; (131): 1–4.

[67] Frenzel JE. Using electronic medical records to teach patient-centered care. Am J Pharm Educ. 2010; 74(4): 71.

[68] Tralongo P, Ferraù F, Borsellino N, Verderame F, Caruso M, et al. Cancer patient-centered home care: a new model for health care in oncology. Ther Clin Risk Manag. 2011; 7: 387–92.

[69] Cooley WC, McAllister JW, Sherrieb K, Clark RE. The medical home index: development and validation of a new practice-level measure of implementation of the medical home model. Ambul Pediatr. 2003; 3(4): 173–80.

[70] Rathert C, Williams ES, McCaughey D, Ishqaidef G. Patient perceptions of patient-centered care: empirical test of a theoretical model. Health Expect. 2012 Available from: http://onlinelibrary.wiley.com/doi/10.1111/hex.12020/pdf. [Accessed 2013-02-28].

[71] VHA Office of Quality and Performance. Survey of Healthcare Experiences of Patients: Methods over view and technical summary. 2009.

[72] Kansagara D, Tuepker A, Joos S, Nicolaidis C, Skaperdas E, Hickman D. Getting performance metrics right: a qualitative study of staff experiences implementing and measuring practice transformation. J Gen Intern Med. 2014; 29(Suppl 2): S607–13.

[73] Christensen EW, Dorrance KA, Ramchandani S, Lynch S, Whitmore CC, et al. Impact of a patient-centered medical home on access, quality, and cost. Mil Med. 2013; 178(2): 135–41.

[74] Henderson S, Princell CO, Martin SD. The patient-centered medical home. Am J Nurs. 2012; 112(12): 54–9.

[75] Rosenberg CN, Peele P, Keyser D, McAnallen S, Holder D. Results from a patient-centered medical home pilot at UPMC health plan hold lessons for broader adoption of the model. Health Aff (Millwood). 2012; 31(11): 2423–31.

[76] Segel S, Hashima J, Gregory WT, Edelman A, Li H, et al. A new approach to postpartum rounds: patient-centered collaborative care improves efficiency. J Grad Med Educ. 2010; 2(1): 67–72.

[77] Nutting PA, Crabtree BF, Stewart EE, Miller WL, Palmer RF, et al. Effect of facilitation on practice outcomes in the national demonstration project model of the patient-centered medical home. Ann Fam Med. 2010; 8(1): 33–4.

[78] Roby DH, Pourat N, Pirritano MJ, Vrungos SM, Dajee H, et al. Impact of patient-centered medical home assignment on emergency room visits among uninsured patients in a county health system. Med Care Res Rev. 2010; 67(4): 412–430.

[79] Steele GD, Haynes JA, Davis DE, Tomcavage J, Stewart WF, et al. How Geisinger's advanced medical home model argues the case for rapid-cycle innovation. Health Aff (Millwood). 2010; 29(11): 2047–53.

[80] Werner RM, Canamucio A, Marcus SC, Terwiesch C. Primary care access and emergency room use among older veterans. J Gen Intern Med. 2014; 29(Suppl 2): 689–94.

[81] Domino ME, Humble C, Lawrence WW Jr, Wegner S. Enhancing the medical homes model for children with asthma. Med Care. 2009; 47: 1113–20.

[82] Peikes D, Chen A, Schore J, Brown R. Effects of care coordination on hospitalization, quality of care, and health care expenditures among Medicare beneficiaries: 15 randomized trials. JAMA. 2009; 301(6): 603–18.

[83] Katz DA, McCoy K, and Sarrazin MV (2014) Does Improved Continuity of Primary Care Affect Clinician–Patient Communication in VA? J Gen Intern Med 29(Suppl 2): S682–8.

[84] Yano EM, Bair MJ, Carrasquillo O, Krein SL, Rubenstein LV. Patient Aligned Care Teams (PACT): VA's journey to implement patient-centered medical homes. J Gen Intern Med. 2014; 29(Suppl 2): S547–9.

[85] Woodward-Hagg H, Workman-Germann J, Flanagan M, Suskovich D, Schachitti S, Corum C, et al. Implementation of Systems Redesign: approaches to spread and sustain adoption. In: Henriksen K, Battles JB, Keyes MA, Grady ML, editors. Advances in patient safety: new directions and alternative approaches (Vol. 2: Culture and Redesign). AGRH (US): 2008.

[86] Rubenstein LV, Stockdale SE, Sapir N, Altman L, Dresselhaus T, et al. A patient-centered primary care practice approach using evidence-based quality improvement: Rationale, methods, and early assessment of implementation. J Gen Intern Med. 2014; 29(Suppl 2): 589–597.

[87] Reid RJ, Wagner EH. The Veterans Health Administration Patient Aligned Care Teams: Lessons in primary care transformation. J Gen Intern Med. 2014; 29(Suppl 2): S552–4.

[88] Bidassie B, Davies ML, Stark R, Boushon B. VA experience in implementing patient-centered medical home using a breakthrough series collaborative. J Gen Intern Med. 2014; 29(Suppl 2): S563–S571.

[89] Institute for Healthcare Improvement. The Breakthrough Series: IHI's collaborative model for achieving breakthrough improvement. 2003.

[90] Davies ML. Systems Redesign Framework for Improvement (TAMMCS). 2009.

[91] Langley GL, Nolan KM, Nolan TW, Norman CL, Provost LP. The Improvement Guide: A Practical Approach to Enhancing Organizational Performance (2nd Edition). Jossey Bass: San Francisco; 2009.

[92] Schectman G, Stark R. Orchestrating large organizational change in primary care: The Veterans' Health Administration experience implementing a patient-centered medical home. J Gen Intern Med. 2014; 29(Suppl 2): S550–1.

[93] Huerta TR, Sieck CJ, Hefner J, Johansen M, Wexler R, et al. Patient centered care plus medical home does not equal patient centered medical home: Why layering models of care may not lead to better outcomes. OA Fam Med. 2013; 1(1): 5.

[94] Goldman RE, Parker DR, Brown J, Walker W, Eaton CB, et al. Recommendations for a mixed methods approach to evaluation the patient-centered medical home. Ann Fam Med. 2015; 13(2): 168–175.

[95] Paustain ML, Alexander JA, El Reda DK, Wise CG, Green LA, et al. Partial and incremental PCMH practice transformation: Implications for quality and costs. Health Serv Res. 2014; 49(1): 52–74.

[96] Ladebue AC, Helfrich CD, Gerdes ZT, Fihn SD, Nelson KM, et al. The experience of Patient Aligned Care Team (PACT) members. Health Care Manage Rev. 2016; 41(1): 2–10.

[97] Helfrich CD, Dolan ED, Simonetti J, Reid RJ, Joos S, et al. Elements of team-based care in a patient-centered medical home are associated with lower burnout among VA primary care employees. J Gen Intern Med. 2014; 29(Suppl 2): S659–66.

[98] Fix GM, Asch SM, Saifu HN, Fletcher MD, Gifford AL, et al. Delivering PACT-principled care: Are specialty care patients being left behind? J Gen Intern Med. 2014; 29(Suppl 2): S695–702.

Chapter 8

Ethical Considerations Related to Narrative Medicine

Halil Tekiner

Additional information is available at the end of the chapter

http://dx.doi.org/10.5772/66167

Abstract

Narrative medicine is of great significance in the area of health care, which underpins the ability of acknowledgment, absorption, and interpretation according to which plights and stories of patients are extensively considered for the commencement of actions. It reflects the manifestation of a model that entails effective medical practice with the aim to achieve best possible outcome. Adopting different approaches to narrative medicine (such as the method of close literature reading and reflective writing) facilitates with the opportunity to examine and explore central medical situations. Narrative medicine is responsible for the development of effective communication between patient and healthcare professionals, alongside inaugurating substantial discourse with the community regarding health care. With the advancement in clinical conditions, the scope of narrative medicine has become a growing need, and thus, several developed countries have already included narrative medicine as an integral part of health care. However, the major ethical problem associated with patient narratives is the use of data with intention other than treatment which may result in maleficence. Therefore, the practice of narrative medicine requires balancing all the aspects of health care against any possible harm.

Keywords: narrative medicine, patient narrative, narrative ethic, ethical concerns, patient-physician relationship

1. Introduction

Patient-centered medicine is an approach that has been greatly integrated into the area of evidence-based medicine and is regarded as an essential attribute underpinned by health care [1, 2]. The description of patient-centered approach put forth by proponents depicts that facilitation of care services in the light of this approach generates numerous opportunities for honoring preferences of the patient, their values, and needs [3]. The patient-centered approach is responsible for applying a biopsychosocial understanding rather than entirely focusing on biomedical knowledge [4]. The major benefit entrenched by the approach is the development of a robust partnership between healthcare professionals and patient [5]. Currently, several studies have covered patient-centered care services and the impacts resulting from it on processes and outcomes of care by extensively emphasizing on the relationship between patient and care facilitators. Nevertheless, much of the patient's experiences result outside the office of a physician [6–8].

Interaction of patients with healthcare professionals has reached beyond the visits to physician's offices through the inclusion of virtual medicine, support from a peer group, and a variety of information as well as the incorporation of communication technologies for the purpose of providing support to care [9]. In addition to this, the ability of a clinician or team of healthcare professionals for the facilitation of patient-centered care is aligned with the setting in which they function (i.e., a small setting for private practices, a large hospital, separate care facility for urgent purposes, or assimilated group practices with multispecialty). On the other hand, the efforts for making the environment of healthcare vigorously responsive to healthcare needs of patients, alongside largely considering their preferences, will assist in the attainment of best possible outcomes if they are encompassed with a profound sense of understanding about the factors through which patient-centered care is promoted or impeded [3, 4]. Moreover, such efforts require a combination of patient-centered care with the system of a healthcare setting as a fundamental property [10].

With the passage of time, a significant shift in medical practices has been observed as a result of tremendous advancements, which, in turn, is improving the quality of life of people around the world. In this regard, narrative medicine has emerged as an essential new set of skills that enhance abilities of healthcare professionals [11]. Narrative medicine is accountable for benefiting healthcare professionals as well as patients with the duration of treatment by providing meaningful ways. The narrative medicine practice has been projected by the aid of a model that entails aspects of reflection, empathy, trust, and professionalism [11]. The basis of narrative competencies is entrenched with the capability of acknowledgment, interpretation of the absorbed information, and acting accordingly to the plights and stories of other individuals [12]. Methods that are entailed with storytelling, reflective writing, and analysis of literature can be utilized for practicing narrative medicine and for the development of narrative competencies. Furthermore, incorporation of narrative medicine approaches in medical education, such as exercises that require illness narrative writings as a method for teaching patient-centeredness, empathy, and humanism of great significance [13].

2. Narrative medicine

Narrative medicine has been developed by a combination of theoretical and operational approaches that have been increasingly applied in the current practices of health care. The existence of this approach is enrooted around 30 years, after which its application has been extensively carried out in daily medical practice as an effective tool for the collection and interpretation of information [11, 14]. The act of clinical method is significantly interpretive that consists of narrative skills for the integration of such stories that overlap with one another and are expressed by patients, healthcare professionals, and test reports. Medical narrative practice aims to comprehend the experience of a patient in regard to his/her feelings and perception about the process [11, 14]. Several scholars have highlighted that listening to the stories shared by a patient is an efficient tool for enriching the knowledge depicting the physical and psychological condition of the patient, alongside offering information that can be utilized for the formulation of diagnosis. Therefore, physicians and other healthcare providers are required to align their daily practices with narrative medicine [10, 11].

Simultaneously, narrative medicine is a descendant that has resulted from the area of literature and medicine, and is parallel to patient-centered care. Medical practice can utilize narrative skills for preserving recognition, absorption, interpretation, and making progress by the help of illness stories told by patients [13]. In addition, narrative medicine, which, in turn, is process-based and interdisciplinary for examining clinical conditions, therapeutic relationship between healthcare professional and patient, and meaning underpinned by health care [15, 16]. The methods of narrative medicine have facilitated with the demonstration that tends to enhance the consistency as well as awareness regarding what other perceives while reducing the level of burnout and fatigue related to compassion [17]. Rapid development in health care has been noted due to extensive implementation of narrative medicine. In several schools of medical practices in the US and Canada, the students have experienced significant improvement in their learning skills by the utilization of narrative methods [18, 19].

The conceptualization of narrative medicine is based on three aspects, which are considered as the foundation of clinical practices. These aspects include investing attentively, representation of facts, and affiliation with the practices and patients. The implementation of these factors provides an opportunity to form an authentic contact between a patient and healthcare professional as a prelude resulted from action. Each of the mentioned factors is combined with in-depth knowledge, competencies, and attitudes for enabling healthcare professionals, their colleagues, as well as patients so that they can undertake the development of effective partnerships on the basis of care and recognition [20].

In context to investing attention, it is regarded as the state that requires a rigorous focus on an individual, written text, or artwork for the purpose of enabling perception without the manifestation of distraction [21]. However, the factor of representation deals with linguistic discussion, which can be put forth in visual form parallel to the formless experience of complex nature for perceiving, reorganizing, and communicating to self and other people involved in the process of care [20]. On the other hand, affiliation is entrenched with a shared commitment and its development by mainly aiming patient's well-being. The attainment of affiliation can be carried out by the formation of meaningful contacts among physicians, patients, and colleagues. The simultaneous implementation of attention and representation leads the participants to sustain affiliation for achieving patient compliance and goals of healing within the clinical practices.

In addition to conceptual factors of narrative medicine on the basis of which the commencement of reflective writing takes place, different types of narratives are integrated according to the clinical condition presented by a patient. In some cases, the situation is also considered for the implementation of a narrative process [22]. For the purpose of facilitating education to healthcare professionals and patients, narratives often play the role of memorable, which, in turn, are formed by experiences for encouraging reflection [13]. The following are some prominent examples regarding different types possessed by narrative medicine.

2.1. Medical interview

Medical interview is the type of narrative medicine which is coined as the most adaptable and beneficial tool for diagnosis and treatment. Conversely, interviewing a patient is also entailed with significant difficulties due to the requirement of physician's active involvement and efficient skills in the area of clinical studies [23]. The demands projected on healthcare professionals are intellectual as well as emotional. The skills to conduct analysis and diagnostic rational must be incorporated in balance, alongside the presence of interpersonal skills for the establishment of patient rapport and the development of better communication with patient [23]. In the area of medical practice, medical interview is responsible for providing an essential pathway for the establishment of an assisting relationship of commitment and trust. The process of observation carried out by verbal and nonverbal means facilitates with important information regarding the patient as an individual. Emotional concerns of the patient are assessed by the aid of behavioral projections of a patient during the interview such as, posture, facial expression, and gesture. In addition to this, the interview consists of face-to-face meeting which either can be video-recorded or audio-recorded [24]. During the interview, the clinical practitioner is able to understand patient's reaction about the manifestation of an illness and how the patient is relating his or herself with others. Another critical element that is widely considered during an interview is the style of communication and behavior of the healthcare professional during the process of interviewing [25].

2.2. Medical history

This type of narrative medicine is underpinned with journal writing that holds medical history and all the aspects related to it, along with the science related to health by keeping the goal of extending the knowledge and understanding of the area. In addition to this, medical history also requires the highest quality of historical studies. Symptoms are included in the medical history, which is reported by the patients or their family members in the form of related medical complaints [26]. The symptoms are then compared to clinical signs; those are determined by directly examining the part described by medical personnel. Conversely, if a patient has a psychiatric condition, then an in-depth and lengthy medical history will be attained, along with a number of details regarding the life and activities of the patient that are relevant to the formulation of an effective plan so that the psychiatric illness can be managed. The information collected through the implementation of this approach, in combination with the physical examination, provides the healthcare professional with a chance to carry out diagnosis and to plan effective treatment [24].

2.3. Literary narratives of patients

The literary narratives provide insight into a diversity possessed by alternative forms and situations associated with medical practices, which tempt the reader to carry out the application of his skills of interpretation for differentiating between obsolescence and tradition [27]. In addition to this, literary patient narratives aid contemporary medicine by providing clarity about tradition, alongside aligning itself with future possibilities that are brought into the present from the past [28]. On the other hand, literary narratives could cause a reduction in valuable evidence of medical practices that vary from those presented by physicians according to their experience [27]. This type of patient narrative assists in reflecting on values entrenched by the clinical events. Some healthcare professional belief that literary narrative is a medium through which readers are provided with a broad vision that develops empathy toward the patient, as well as compassion for serving human and enhancing sense of ethics [29].

2.4. Classical illness narratives

Patient stories allow healthcare professionals to understand the sufferings and feelings experienced by the patients and their family members. These stories are presented by combining biographical context with the social context of the clinical condition for the purpose of suggesting strategies to cope. These narratives are of great potential for assisting a person with personal development [30].

2.5. Patient-physician narratives

Patient-physician narratives are articulated and formed by obtaining information about the illness, and the process associated with the condition. The experience of patients regarding the clinical symptoms is then interpreted by the utilization of medical knowledge possessed by the involved healthcare practitioners, which, in turn, lead to an efficient diagnosis and therapeutic intervention [31]. After the diagnosis of the condition, the narrative of the patient changes about their personal experience, as the perception of medical diagnosis and therapeutics plays a major role on their sensations. This type of narrative is frequently used during the treatment of cancer [32, 33].

3. Expected outcomes of narrative medicine

A narrative is entrenched with the potential for informing, revealing, healing, and inspiring through different ways, which help in the dissemination of best possible outcomes [14, 34]. With the addition of a human lens, experiences related to health care are enriched, without causing detraction of the important facts and time frames [35]. Similar to their patients, some of the healthcare practitioners have involved in the process of learning so that they can effectively attain help for verbal representation about they experience throughout their medical practices. Several physicians write narratives about their practices for keeping records about how they interact with other people. Narratives help the doctors to illustrate aspects related to their emotions and personality and the care they provide to their patients. Some of the authors have reported that narrative writings have helped them in comprehending the ordeals associated with their patients by aligning their lives with the people who have disease [35, 36].

The utilization of narratives entailing healthcare professionals, stories of patients, film, and literature is extensively gaining popularity in the area of medical education. However, there is a profound need to encompass conceptual framework so that these efforts can be provided with significant guidance in curricula of medical schools [19]. Through interpreting their observations, the doctors, who are also the writers of patient narratives, can unveil great truths that are encompassed by the illness course regarding an ordinary life of a person. Dr. Rita Charon, a director of the Narrative Medicine Program at the Columbia University College of Physicians and Surgeons and a clinical medicine professor, is well known for her immense contribution in the area of narrative medicine. Dr. Charon described that there is a profound need of physicians by the people who are presented with a clinical condition [11, 14]. The underlying reason for such need is that physicians are able to understand the disease and facilitate with high quality care services. People have a perception that reflects physicians not only provide treatment of their illness, but also accompany their patients throughout the course of treatment [11]. On the other hand, utilization of patient narrative for designing healthcare services, to conduct research, or for providing medical education, is encompassed with both pros and cons. Therefore, significant consideration is required by keeping rules and regulation in mind before using patient narratives for the stated purposes [37]. Following are some of the major pros and cons associated with the patient narratives.

3.1. Pros of patient narrative

1. The method of the patient narrative is significantly conventional due to which the implementation of such approach is extensively practiced [21].

2. The method underpins great aspects of flexibility and can be utilized in several clinical settings [21].

3. Nurses can also record the chronological events related to a situation through the use of this system [38].

4. The narrative type of documentation provides assistance to the healthcare professionals by painting a picture that elaborates care services facilitated to a patient for an extended duration [21].

5. Patient narratives can be easily used in emergency situations due to the aspect of quick charting [38].

6. Patient narratives can be easily integrated with other methods of documentation (i.e., flow sheets) [21].

7. Patient narratives provide significant opportunity to develop logic and motivations regarding patient's condition that otherwise appear irrelevant [39].

3.2. Cons of patient narrative

1. The notes taken in the form of patient narratives depict subjectivity and the approach also lack nursing evidence related to analysis that plays an important role in the decision-making process [26].

2. Significant limitations can be noticed in patient narratives, which entail perceptions and perspectives [38].

3. Patient narrative notes are not structured and are often presented in a disorganized form without any continuity [40].

4. Scanning notes may consume time for searching fundamental information depending on the feature of disorganization [41].

5. These notes can be considered as task oriented, alongside incorporating less or no focus on evaluation [26].

6. Healthcare professionals are often encountered with frustration at the time of tracking a particular aspect associated with the condition of a patient [41].

7. Patient narratives may be difficult for keeping the track of patient's condition and progress due to several documentation processes carried out by various healthcare practitioners on different days or shifts for registering the similar event [26].

The skills required to use narratives in healthcare practices are of great importance. In this context, teaching methods have been designed to prepare efficient practitioners. Some of the prominent medical education programs have been assimilated in "narrative medicine" or "narrative-based medicine" for the purpose of teaching particular aspects embedded by narrative competence [18, 19]. The mentioned type of educational training tends to encourage healthcare practitioners as well as students by improving their writing skills through the use of a nontechnical language so that they can keep the record of their patient's condition [22]. In addition to this, patient narratives are also widely used by healthcare patients for attaining help so that they can disclose and understand their state of mind toward their patient's condition. The importance of narrative medicine programs can be evaluated from the fact that they promote rigorous training through which the learners appropriately encounter how to read literary texts for further supplying healthcare professionals with the interpretative tool, alongside creating a sense of the patient's stories. At some occasion, healthcare practitioners provide encouragement to their patients for describing their condition in the form of a written text. The narratives were written by patient project significant interruption of the text flow and assist the healthcare professionals in demonstrating therapeutic benefits associated with the narration to the patient [42].

Narrative medicine curricula and projects have been proliferating throughout the US, Great Britain,Canada, Europe, and Australia [43]. In the US, the narrative medicine study is regarded as the multidisciplinary area, while the master's program curriculum of narrative medicine embeds fundamental courses that are responsible for providing the students with an in-depth understanding of the experiences related illness, the equipment for closely reading and writing [44]. On the other hand, focused narrative courses are used in the areas such as genetics, palliative care, social justice advocacy, and field work. The narrative medicine study provided in Great Britain emphasizes on the investigation of patient stories for understanding symptoms and experiences of the patient in case reports and clinical literature. The medical narrative students are trained to comprehend interfaces related to descriptions and images, such as the textual presentation of a disease, text written by a patient, and diagnosis resulting from close reading [35].

The educational programs of narrative medicine in Canada enhance the ability of learners to apply best practices by analyzing the principles deep-rooted by narrative, alongside the manifestation of arts-based research in the area of health care. The educational programs encourage the students to carry out utilization of their investigative and interpretive skills that are required for closely reading, actively listening, visual literacy, and reflective writing for enhancing diagnosis and therapy [45].

Regarding the narrative medicine programs in Australia, the area of education is making a tremendous progress by dispersing awareness among current and future healthcare professionals about the impacts of narrative medicine in practice. The master's program of narrative medicine strengthens the attainment of best possible outcomes in several fields, including medicine, social justice, public health, and clinical experiences of an individual [18].

4. Challenges of narrative medicine

An approach of narrative medicine plays a vital role in facilitation of healthcare services. The rapid evolution of modern medicine tends to contribute to the challenges posed to narrative medicine due to the requirement of profound attitudinal and technical modifications. These changes are of great significance and are difficult to apply. During its initial stages, the practices of narrative medicine can be converted into a destabilization phase, which, in turn, position a capable healthcare practitioner in doubt about his or her practices [46]. Another major challenge that can be encountered during the integration of narrative medicine include is acknowledging when to discontinue. Healthcare practitioners who closely associated themselves with the notion of narratives often forget to realize that their position is not safe [46].

5. Ethical concerns

The ethics required for medical narratives are considered as the act of evaluating language that is aligned with perceptions, thoughts, and sensations experienced by the teller so that others can relate to what he or she is trying to describe [14]. The individual who receives narrative of another person also receives virtue of the teller, which, in turn, plays the role of an intersubjective bridge to the ethics of narrative medicine. On the other hand, the major ethical problem associated with patient narratives is the use of data with intention other than treatment which may result in maleficence [14]. In today's world of technological development, narrative ethics and non-maleficence require balancing all the aspects of health care against any possible harm [47].

Although narrative medicine has emerged as ubiquitously identified the domain of study, the manifestation of ethical concerns reflecting maintained of privacy and confidentiality of patient's data has raised several questions [12]. The study of Nelson depicts that the framework of medical ethics is regarded as an essential part of an individual's professional identification, instead of projecting skills and knowledge. Simultaneously, the critical aspects underpinned by the identity of a healthcare professional are operating within the formal prospects in more subtle way. The authors also stated that education and use of narrative medicine are responsible for establishing "moral enculturation," which possesses a subtle part of formal teachings of ethics [48]. Moreover, any attempt that is put forth for the development of comprehensive syllabus of ethics must allow the manifestation of wider setting of different cultures within which the syllabus must be implemented. For the purpose of fostering ethics among students, formal as well as informal syllabus must be addressed through the aid of syllabus planners. However, Goldie states that without an adequate consideration, physicians may be in danger of objectifying and manipulating patients in accordance with an egocentric self-interest [49].

The current form of narrative medicine provides a small space for aligning the properties of critical reflection or examination of larger inequities and violence. The violence is of structural nature that takes place within a healthcare setting in the light of which feelings of people are neglected. Marini illustrates that narrative medicine lacks consideration of the narrative limits, particularly ignoring the contexts related to suffering, trauma, and oppression. In other words, people are often bounded by certain experiences due to which their assimilation with the storyline does not match. Experiences gained by a human cannot be narrated in a single story as a result of which gesture and metaphor can be integrated as an effective means for the development of better communication between patient and healthcare professional [26].

Of course, confidentiality protections play a fundamental role in the practices of patient narratives for patients and people who are involved in the process of writing. In this context, a number of questions have been raised such as, does patient narrative lead to the promotion of new learning and self-understanding or is it the procedural intention toward self-justification? [20]. However, regarding the ethical concerns, the practices of patient narratives entail alteration or removal of personal data through which an individual can be identified. Several healthcare professionals have encountered resistance from patient as they fear that their personal information could be used for other purposes or personal benefits of the healthcare settings [48]. The pitfall of data breaching is assured by several national regulations (i.e., Health Insurance Portability and Accountability Act) [50]. On the other hand, the International Conference on Harmonization (ICH) has proposed a set of guidelines regarding the content and structure of patient narratives. According to their guidelines, it is mandatory to provide an explanation of possible adverse events or other adverse effects that can be investigated for clinical importance [22].

The notion of ethical concerns related to patient narratives is responsible for contributing to complications in decision-making process, which is the essential step in designing a treatment plan. It is necessary for the healthcare professionals to maintain significant balance between narratives of patient and their decisions [14]. Simultaneously, narrative is presented with the requirement of developing a relationship of confidentiality through respecting privacy of patients so that they can be encouraged to seek care services. For the purpose of sustaining confidentiality, the obligation associated with it prohibits disclosure of the patient's information presented in a narrative form [51].

6. Discussion and result

Narrative medicine is largely utilized in health care for the promotion of the integrated, systemic, and multidisciplinary development of an approach through which populations can be facilitated with care, regardless of their age groups [11, 14]. The stories illustrated by patients and healthcare professionals, along with their way of representing, perceiving, and experiencing can lead to the reduction in the risk associated with inappropriate clinical tests and treatments [14]. The area of health care has always been encountered with significant saturation, alongside the presence of narrative knowledge. Over the past few decades, an increase assimilation of writing into research and teaching has been observed in the form of narrative medicine [19, 23, 45]. In addition to this, the most commonly occurring ethical concerns is encompassed with barriers and uncertainties associated with truth elaborating, along with cultural and familial conflict, as well as futility [40]. In this regard, physicians and other practitioners' function by offering strategies to develop effective communication with patients and their family members.

In the context of the current practices of narrative medicine, different types of narratives are incorporating the power of appreciation and analysis in the clinical studies by the aid of storytelling [43]. Team of healthcare professionals is at the forefront for facilitating with information based on prognosis. Shortly, narrative medicine would be able to separate its root from assumptions and methods utilized during the process of history taking as well as for eliminating the possibility of several conflicts. Medical practitioners and educators are gradually including many approaches and techniques that are underpinned by literary studies, philosophy, history, along with other disciplines of humanities for bridging the gap that projects a lack of recognition and understanding a particular illness and the pathological dimension associated with it. However, there is a profound need of educating students of narrative medicine about potential ethical concerns, which can lead to negative outcomes of health. Ethical concerns mostly deal with information breaching as a result of which several patients avoid to participate in the process of narrative writing. Therefore, it is the fundamental responsibility of the healthcare practitioners to develop a therapeutic relationship with their patients so that the flow of information can be maintained [40, 47, 48, 52].

Narrative medicine has contributed greatly by aligning trustworthiness and compassion with medical ethics. Competency of practicing narrative medicine and a framework of narrative for medical ethics can lead to the enhancement of ethical considerations at various stages including recognizing an ethical issue, oral or written form of the issue, ethical case interpretation, and selected interpretation with its validation. Ideally, narrative medicine would assist healthcare professionals in the prevention of ethical dilemmas by increasing the chances of recognizing the issue at its initial stage and resolving it [40, 49].

Narrative medicine should be explored more deeply to decode techniques through which clinical conversations can be shaped. The noticeable proliferation of writings in the past years has emanated a new perceptive of health as well as social care and different situations associated with it. The narrative medicine not only sheds light on metaphors possessed by various clinical conditions but also provides direction to imagery presentation of diseases in a graphic novel and films. The best possible health outcomes are obtained when health care and social work are combined with ethical narrative medicine practice. The resultant of narrative medicine is capable of eliciting and functioning with illness stories and worlds depicting the fractured life of a person by acknowledging the importance of communication through telling and listening to stories [11, 14, 40, 53].

Acknowledgements

The author wishes to cordially thank Dr. Hale Zerrin Toklu for critically proof-reading this chapter.

Author details

Halil Tekiner*

Address all correspondence to: htekiner@erciyes.edu.tr

Erciyes University Faculty of Pharmacy, Department of Pharmaceutical History and Ethics, Melikgazi, Kayseri, Turkey

References

[1] Phelan M, Stradins L, Morrison S. Towards a global definition of patient centred care. Psychiatry. 1998;155:974–976

[2] Sackett DL, Rosenberg WMC, Gray JAM, Haynes RB, Richardson WS. Evidence based medicine: what it is and what it isn't. BMJ. 1996;312(7023):71–72

[3] Epstein RM, Street RL, Jr. The values and value of patient-centered care. Ann Fam Med. 2011;9(2):100–103. doi:10.1370/afm.1239

[4] Constand MK, MacDermid JC, Dal Bello-Haas V, Law M. Scoping review of patient-centered care approaches in healthcare. BMC Health Serv Res. 2014;14(1):271. doi: 10.1186/1472-6963-14-271

[5] Toklu HZ. Promoting evidence-based practice in pharmacies. Integr Pharm Res Pract. 2015;4:127–131. doi:10.2147/IPRP.S70406

[6] Epstein RM. The science of patient-centered care. J Fam Pract. 2000;49(9): 805–807

[7] Greene SM, Tuzzio L, Cherkin D. A framework for making patient-centered care front and center. Perm J. 2012;16(3):49–53

[8] Stewart M, Brown JB, Donner A, McWhinney IR, Oates J, Weston WW, et al. The impact of patient-centered care on outcomes. J Fam Pract. 2000;49(9):796–804

[9] Kelley JM, Kraft-Todd G, Schapira L, Kossowsky J, Riess H. The influence of the patient-clinician relationship on healthcare outcomes: a systematic review and meta-analysis of randomized controlled trials. PLoS One. 2014;9(4):e94207. doi:10.1371/journal.pone.0094207

[10] Peabody FW. The care of the patient. JAMA. 2015;313(18):1868. doi:10.1001/jama.2014.11744

[11] Charon R. The patient-physician relationship. Narrative medicine: a model for empathy, reflection, profession, and trust. JAMA. 2001;286(15):1897–1902. doi:10.1001/jama.286.15.1897

[12] Zhou C, Wu Y, An S, Li X. Effect of expressive writing intervention on health outcomes in breast cancer patients: a systematic review and meta-analysis of randomized controlled trials. PLoS One. 2015;10(7):e0131802. doi:10.1371/journal.pone.0131802

[13] Blickem C, Priyadharshini E. Patient narratives: the potential for "patient-centred" interprofessional learning? J Interprof Care. 2007;21(6):619–632. doi:10.1080/13561820701653482

[14] Charon R. Narrative Medicine: Honoring the Stories of Illness. Oxford: Oxford University Press; 2008

[15] Nowaczyk MJ. Narrative medicine in clinical genetics practice. Am J Med Genet. 2012;158(8):1941–1947. doi:10.1002/ajmg.a.35482

[16] Roberts A, Gaizauskas R, Hepple M, Guo Y. Mining clinical relationships from patient narratives. BMC Bioinformatics. 2008;11:S3. doi:10.1186/1471-2105-9-S11-S3

[17] Fioretti C, Mazzocco K, Riva S, Oliveri S, Masiero M, Pravettoni G. Research studies on patients' illness experience using the narrative medicine approach: a systematic review. BMJ Open. 2016;6(7):e011220

[18] Arntfield SL, Slesar K, Dickson J, Charon R. Narrative medicine as a means of training medical students toward residency competencies. Patient Educ Couns. 2013;91(3):280–286. doi:10.1016/j.pec.2013.01.014

[19] Kumagai AK. A conceptual framework for the use of illness narratives in medical education. Acad Med. 2008;83(7):653–658. doi:10.1097/acm.0b013e3181782e17

[20] Di Gangi S, Naretto G, Cravero N, Livigni S. A narrative-based study on communication by family members in intensive care unit. J Crit Care. 2013;28(4):483–489. doi:10.1016/j.jcrc.2012.11.001

[21] Smorti A, Fioretti C. Why narrating changes memory: a contribution to an integrative model of memory and narrative processes. Integr Psychol Behav Sci. 2016;50(2):296–319. doi:10.1007/s12124-015-9330-6

[22] Kulkarni NG, Dalal JJ, Kulkarni TN. Audio-video recording of informed consent process: Boon or bane. Perspect Clin Res. 2014;5(1):6–10. doi:10.4103/2229-3485.124547

[23] Wear D, Zarconi J, Garden R, Jones T. Reflection in/and writing: pedagogy and practice in medical education. Acad Med. 2012;87(5):603–609. doi:10.1097/ACM.0b013e31824d22e9

[24] Hess DW, Reed VA, Turco MG, Parboosingh JT, Bernstein HH. Enhancing provider engagement in practice improvement: a conceptual framework. J Contin Educ Health Prof. 2015;35(1):71–79. doi:10.1002/chp.21260

[25] Greenfield BH, Jensen GM, Delany CM, Mostrom E, Knab M, Jampel A. Power and promise of narrative for advancing physical therapist education and practice. Phys Ther. 2015;95(6):924–933. doi:10.2522/ptj.20140085

[26] Marini MG. Bridging the gap between personalization of care and research. In: Marini MG, editor. Narrative Medicine. New York: Springer; 2016. pp. 59–69

[27] Kottow M, Kottow A. Literary narrative in medical practice. Med Humanit. 2002;28(1):41–44. doi:10.1136/mh.28.1.41

[28] Bleakley A. Medical Humanities and Medical Education: How the Medical Humanities Can Shape Better Doctors. New York: Routledge; 2015

[29] Bury M. Illness narratives: fact or fiction? Sociol Health Ill. 2001;23(3):263–285. doi:10.1111/1467-9566.00252

[30] Fioretti C, Smorti A. Narrating positive versus negative memories of illness: does narrating influence the availability and the emotional involvement of memories of illness. Eur J Cancer Care. doi:10.1111/ecc.12524

[31] Jurecic A. Illness as Narrative. Pittsburgh: University of Pittsburgh Press; 2012

[32] Hunt L. Strategic suffering: illness narratives as social empowerment among Mexican cancer patients. In: Mattingly C, Garro LC, editors. Narrative and the Cultural Construction of Illness and Healing. Berkeley: University of California Press; 2000. pp. 88–107

[33] Salander P. Bad news from the patient's perspective: an analysis of the written narratives of newly diagnosed cancer patients. Soc Sci Med. 2002;55(5):721–732. doi:10.1016/S0959-8049(01)81356-3

[34] Cepeda MS, Chapman CR, Miranda N, Sanchez R, Rodriguez CH, Restrepo AE, et al. Emotional disclosure through patient narrative may improve pain and well-being: results of a randomized controlled trial in patients with cancer pain. J Pain Symptom Manage. 2008;35(6):623–631. doi:10.1016/j.jpainsymman.2007.08.011

[35] Miller E, Balmer D, Hermann N, Graham G, Charon R. Sounding narrative medicine: studying students' professional identity development at Columbia University College of Physicians and Surgeons. Acad Med. 2014;89(2):335–342. doi:10.1097/acm.0000000000000098

[36] Sørlie V, Lindseth A, Udén G, Norberg A. Women physicians' narratives about being in ethically difficult care situations in paediatrics. Nurs Ethics. 2000;7(1):47–62. doi:10.1177/096973300000700107

[37] Broom B. Naming what we do. EJPCH. 2016;4(2):265–270. doi:10.5750/ejpch.v4i2.1200

[38] Iyer PW. Nursing Malpractice. Tucson: Lawyers & Judges Publishing Company; 2001

[39] DeLaune SC, Ladner PK. Nursing Fundamentals: Standards & Practice. Singapore: Cengage Learning; 2011

[40] Charon R. Narrative medicine: form, function, and ethics. Ann Intern Med. 2001;134(1):83–87. doi:10.7326/0003-4819-134-1-200101020-00024

[41] Prideaux A. Issues in nursing documentation and record-keeping practice. Br J Nurs. 2011;20(22):1450–1454. doi:10.12968/bjon.2011.20.22.1450

[42] Murphy JW. Primary health care and narrative medicine. Perm J. 2015;19(4):90–94. doi:10.7812/TPP/14-206

[43] Charon R. What to do with stories: the sciences of narrative medicine. Can Fam Physician. 2007;53(8):1265–1267

[44] Rider EA, Kurtz S, Slade D, Longmaid HE, Ho MJ, Pun JK, et al. The International Charter for Human Values in Healthcare: an interprofessional global collaboration to enhance values and communication in healthcare. Patient Educ Couns. 2014;96(3):273–280. doi:10.1016/j.pec.2014.06.017

[45] Bhavaraju VL, Miller S. Faculty development in narrative medicine: using stories to teach, learn, and thrive. J Grad Med Educ. 2014;6(2):355–356. doi:10.4300/jgme-d-14-00077

[46] Kalitzkus V, Matthiessen PF. Narrative-based medicine: potential, pitfalls, and practice. Perm J. 2009;13(1):80–86

[47] Beauchamp TL, Childress JF. Principles of Biomedical Ethics. Oxford: Oxford University Press; 2001

[48] Nelson HL. Stories and Their Limits: Narrative Approaches to Bioethics. New York: Routledge; 2014

[49] Goldie JGS. The ethics of listening and responding to patients' narratives: implications for practice. Br J Gen Pract. 2011;61(585):306–307. doi:10.3399/bjgp11X568143

[50] Annas GJ. HIPAA regulations: a new era of medical-record privacy? NEJM. 2003;348(15):1486–1490. doi:10.1056/nejmlim035027

[51] Hooker C. Ethics and the arts in the medical humanities. In: Macneill P, editor. Ethics and the Arts. Dordrecht: Springer; 2014. pp. 213–224

[52] Brody H. My story is broken; can you help me fix it? Medical ethics and the joint construction of narrative. Lit Med. 1994;13(1):79–92. doi:10.1353/lm.2011.0169

[53] Charon R. At the membranes of care: stories in narrative medicine. Acad Med. 2012;87(3):342–347. doi:10.1097/acm.0b013e3182446fbb